Handbook of
FISH DISEASES

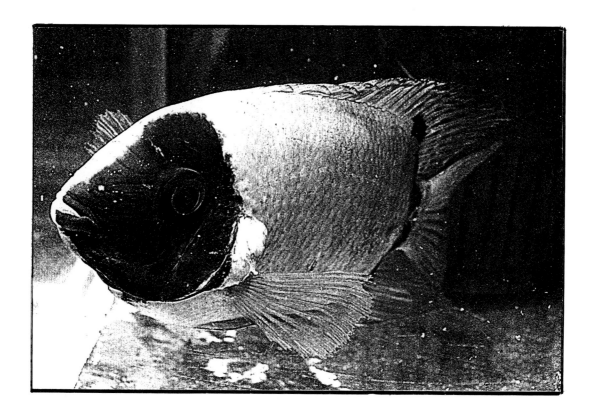

DIETER UNTERGASSER
Translated by Howard H. Hirschhorn

Edited for the English-language market by
Dr. Herbert R. Axelrod

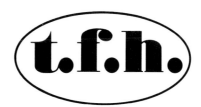

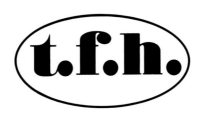

© 1989 by T.F.H. Publications, Inc.

Distributed in the UNITED STATES by T.F.H. Publications, Inc., One T.F.H. Plaza, Neptune City, NJ 07753; in CANADA to the Pet Trade by H & L Pet Supplies Inc., 27 Kingston Crescent, Kitchener, Ontario N2B 2T6; Rolf C. Hagen Ltd., 3225 Sartelon Street, Montreal 382 Quebec; in CANADA to the Book Trade by Macmillan of Canada (A Division of Canada Publishing Corporation), 164 Commander Boulevard, Agincourt, Ontario M1S 3C7; in ENGLAND by T.F.H. Publications Limited, Cliveden House/Priors Way/Bray, Maidenhead, Berkshire SL6 2HP, England; in AUSTRALIA AND THE SOUTH PACIFIC by T.F.H. (Australia) Pty. Ltd., Box 149, Brookvale 2100 N.S.W., Australia; in NEW ZEALAND by Ross Haines & Son, Ltd., 18 Monmouth Street, Grey Lynn, Auckland 2, New Zealand; in the PHILIPPINES by Bio-Research, 5 Lippay Street, San Lorenzo Village, Makati Rizal; in SOUTH AFRICA by Multipet Pty. Ltd., 30 Turners Avenue, Durban 4001. Published by T.F.H. Publications, Inc. Manufactured in the United States of America by T.F.H. Publications, Inc.

Contents

NOTE BY EDITOR OF ENGLISH-LANGUAGE EDITION

This is, without a doubt, the finest book on diseases of aquarium fishes ever of-
fered to aquarists. The excellent photographic skills of the author, Dieter Untergasser, coupled with his organized approach to the subject, make it easily possible for a major change in the quality of aquarium fishes sold in petshops
worldwide. For once a serious aquarium shop owner can easily evaluate the
quality (health-wise) of the fishes he has purchased, recognize and identify fish
diseases, and properly treat them. This book can also serve the serious hobbyist.
Never before has a step-by-step book in fish pathology ever been attempted.

Because of the high regard I have for this book, I put a lot of effort into it. I also
had some problems. Almost all of the drugs recommended by the author were
of German origin and had German names. I had to find their English, American,
Australian, etc., equivalents and put them into the book. The same was true of
much of the equipment, techniques, procedures, protocols and measurements.

I left in the metric system. If you don't have a good grasp of the metric system
you can refer to the Measurement Conversion Factors section that I have in-
cluded on page 6.

The decimal system the author uses is simple and easy to understand. A problem arose with the translation of the word we would use for 'illustration.' We didn't
want a separate numbering system for photos and drawings . . . so, there being
so few drawings, we decided to name all the illustrations 'photograph' . . . don't
be upset by seeing a drawing called a photograph . . . at least it enabled me to
put all the illustrations in sequential order.

I added to the book the PHARMACOPOEIA. This was enhanced with a "Where
to buy it" reference wherever possible.

If you're looking for a book that puts fish disease recognition, treatment and
prevention onto a truly systematic and understandable basis, I know you will enjoy this book as much as I do.

Dr. Herbert R. Axelrod

Acknowledgments

My wife Helga deserves many thanks for her understanding and moral support during the writing of this book. I also thank Mr. Bauer, formerly of Hohenheim University, for the systematic organization of the gill worms (Dactylogyridea) and the nematodes (Oxyurida). In addition, I would like to thank the many aquarium owners and breeders who often went out of their way to bring me diseased specimens.

Measurement Conversion Factors

When you know—	Multiply by—	To find—
Length:		
Millimeters (mm)	0.04	inches (in)
Centimeters (cm)	0.4	inches (in)
Meters (m)	3.3	feet (ft)
Meters (m)	1.1	yards (yd)
Kilometers (km)	0.6	miles (mi)
Inches (in)	2.54	centimeters (cm)
Feet (ft)	30	centimeters (cm)
Yards (yd)	0.9	meters (m)
Miles (mi)	1.6	kilometers (km)
Area:		
Square centimeters (cm^2)	0.16	square inches (sq in)
Square meters (m^2)	1.2	square yards (sq yd)
Square kilometers (km^2)	0.4	square miles (sq mi)
Hectares (ha)	2.5	acres
Square inches (sq in)	6.5	square centimeters (cm^2)
Square feet (sq ft)	0.09	square meters (m^2)
Square yards (sq yd)	0.8	square meters (m^2)
Square miles (sq mi)	1.2	square kilometers (km^2)
Acres	0.4	hectares (ha)
Mass (Weight):		
Grams (g)	0.035	ounces (oz)
Kilograms (kg)	2.2	pounds (lb)
Ounces (oz)	28	grams (g)
Pounds (lb)	0.45	kilograms (kg)
Volume:		
Milliliters (ml)	0.03	fluid ounces (fl oz)
Liters (L)	2.1	pints (pt)
Liters (L)	1.06	quarts (qt)
Liters (L)	0.26	U.S. gallons (gal)
Liters (L)	0.22	Imperial gallons (gal)
Cubic centimeters (cc)	16.387	cubic inches (cu in)
Cubic meters (cm^3)	35	cubic feet (cu ft)
Cubic meters (cm^3)	1.3	cubic yards (cu yd)
Teaspoons (tsp)	5	millimeters (ml)
Tablespoons (tbsp)	15	millimeters (ml)
Fluid ounces (fl oz)	30	millimeters (ml)
Cups (c)	0.24	liters (L)
Pints (pt)	0.47	liters (L)
Quarts (qt)	0.95	liters (L)
U.S. gallons (gal)	3.8	liters (L)
U.S. gallons (gal)	231	cubic inches (cu in)
Imperial gallons (gal)	4.5	liters (L)
Imperial gallons (gal)	277.42	cubic inches (cu in)
Cubic inches (cu in)	0.061	cubic centimeters (cc)
Cubic feet (cu ft)	0.028	cubic meters (m^3)
Cubic yards (cu yd)	0.76	cubic meters (m^3)
Temperature:		
Celsius (°C)	multiply by 1.8, add 32	Fahrenheit (°F)
Fahrenheit (°F)	subtract 32, multiply by 0.555	Celsius (°C)

Introduction

To offer your fish a healthy "environment encased in glass" presupposes a certain understanding of their behavior and of the biological and chemical factors that affect them both in their natural habitat and in the aquarium. The home aquarium is a "piece of portable nature" only to a limited extent; it should rather be considered as an artificial—and even also artfully arranged—garden.

Most aquarium fish come from the tropics, where they live in extremely clean waters with low conductivity and hardness, high oxygen content, and often with many dissolved organic substances. Today, while it is quite possible to chemically adjust aquarium water to match the fish's natural waters, it is hardly possible to approach their degree of cleanliness. That is simply because of the very small volume of aquarium water. In nature a fish has huge quantities of water in which to feed and leave its droppings. In the aquarium, however, fecal dilution is quite limited. The more the fish swims in the aquarium, the more burdened or polluted the water becomes. Polluted water, in turn, harbors microorganisms that are harmful to the fish. Many of these organisms are bacteria and fungi that normally live on the bottom of the tank or in the water, but they also can cause disease. In the wild, where the fish lives in large quantities of water, it is not often confronted with such organisms. The fish can easily ward off an infection. In the closed system of an aquarium, however, the disease-causing organisms multiply. The fish is constantly picking them up, and its body, to a certain extent, is continually attempting to stop these organisms from multiplying in and on it. The fish easily succeeds in resisting them if it is fed well and if it feels at home in its aquarium— and that involves proper water quality and landscaping.

With good hygiene, you can make it tough for the disease-causing organisms to survive. Immediately remove any dead or sick fish. Regularly vacuum out any accumulations of debris from the bottom crevices and from the nooks and crannies of any decorative items in the landscaping. The bacterial count in the water can be significantly lowered by use of an ultraviolet lamp in the filter reflux.

Just as in waters in the wild, the aquarium also has a biological self-cleansing cycle. You must recognize and foster this process in order to effectively care for the water in an aquarium, for, as indicated above, it has a direct relationship with the health of the fish. There are many books on water chemistry and aquarium hygiene. The better this process of self-cleansing is achieved—keeping the water quality high for longer periods— the rarer will be diseases in the aquarium.

Books on the subject allow the interested hobbyist to independently yet effectively increase his knowledge of aquariums, biology, fish pathology, parasitology, and microscopy.

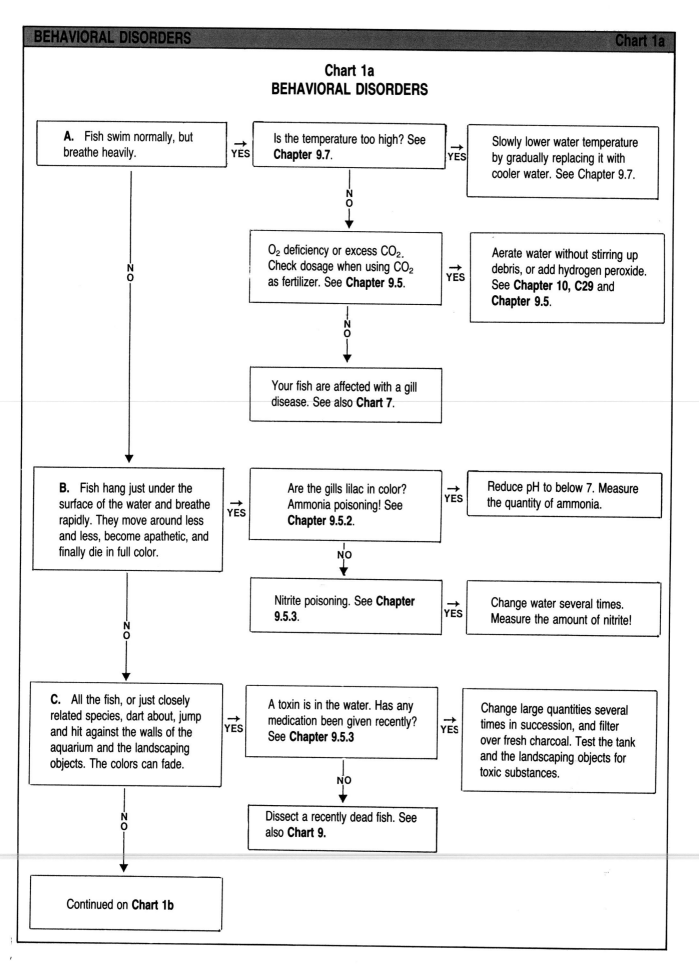

Chart 1a
BEHAVIORAL DISORDERS

A. Fish swim normally, but breathe heavily.

→ YES → Is the temperature too high? See **Chapter 9.7**.

→ YES → Slowly lower water temperature by gradually replacing it with cooler water. See Chapter 9.7.

NO ↓

O_2 deficiency or excess CO_2. Check dosage when using CO_2 as fertilizer. See **Chapter 9.5**.

→ YES → Aerate water without stirring up debris, or add hydrogen peroxide. See **Chapter 10, C29** and **Chapter 9.5**.

NO ↓

Your fish are affected with a gill disease. See also **Chart 7**.

B. Fish hang just under the surface of the water and breathe rapidly. They move around less and less, become apathetic, and finally die in full color.

→ YES → Are the gills lilac in color? Ammonia poisoning! See **Chapter 9.5.2**.

→ YES → Reduce pH to below 7. Measure the quantity of ammonia.

NO ↓

Nitrite poisoning. See **Chapter 9.5.3**.

→ YES → Change water several times. Measure the amount of nitrite!

C. All the fish, or just closely related species, dart about, jump and hit against the walls of the aquarium and the landscaping objects. The colors can fade.

→ YES → A toxin is in the water. Has any medication been given recently? See **Chapter 9.5.3**

→ YES → Change large quantities several times in succession, and filter over fresh charcoal. Test the tank and the landscaping objects for toxic substances.

NO ↓

Dissect a recently dead fish. See also **Chart 9**.

NO ↓

Continued on **Chart 1b**

Chart 1b
Behavioral Disorders (continued)

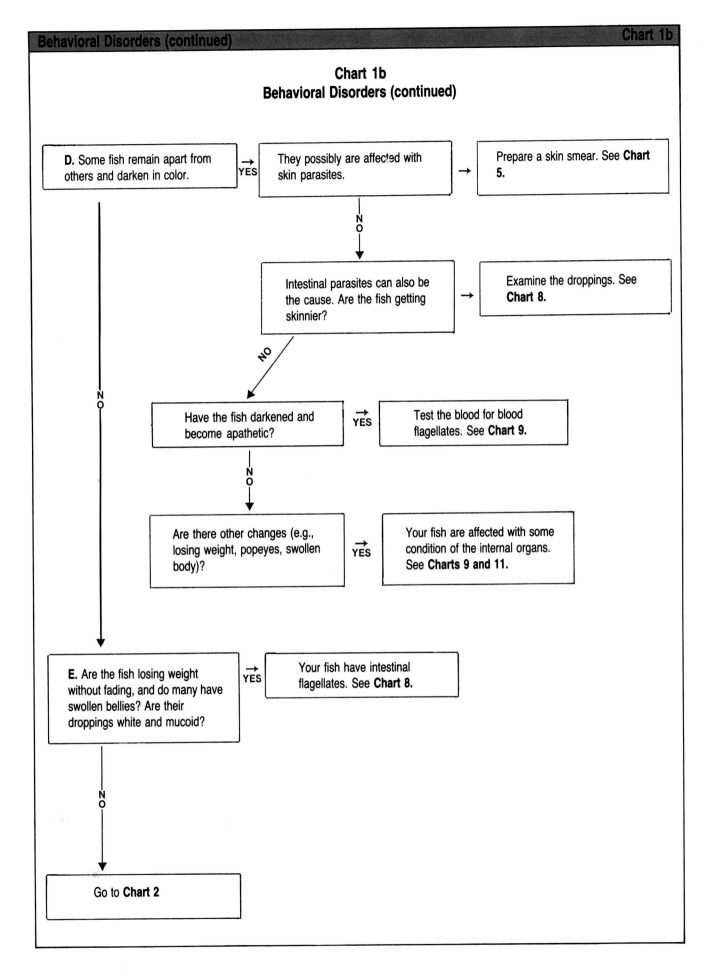

D. Some fish remain apart from others and darken in color.

→ YES

They possibly are affected with skin parasites.

→ Prepare a skin smear. See **Chart 5.**

NO

Intestinal parasites can also be the cause. Are the fish getting skinnier?

→ Examine the droppings. See **Chart 8.**

NO

Have the fish darkened and become apathetic?

→ YES Test the blood for blood flagellates. See **Chart 9.**

NO

Are there other changes (e.g., losing weight, popeyes, swollen body)?

→ YES Your fish are affected with some condition of the internal organs. See **Charts 9 and 11.**

NO

E. Are the fish losing weight without fading, and do many have swollen bellies? Are their droppings white and mucoid?

→ YES Your fish have intestinal flagellates. See **Chart 8.**

NO

Go to **Chart 2**

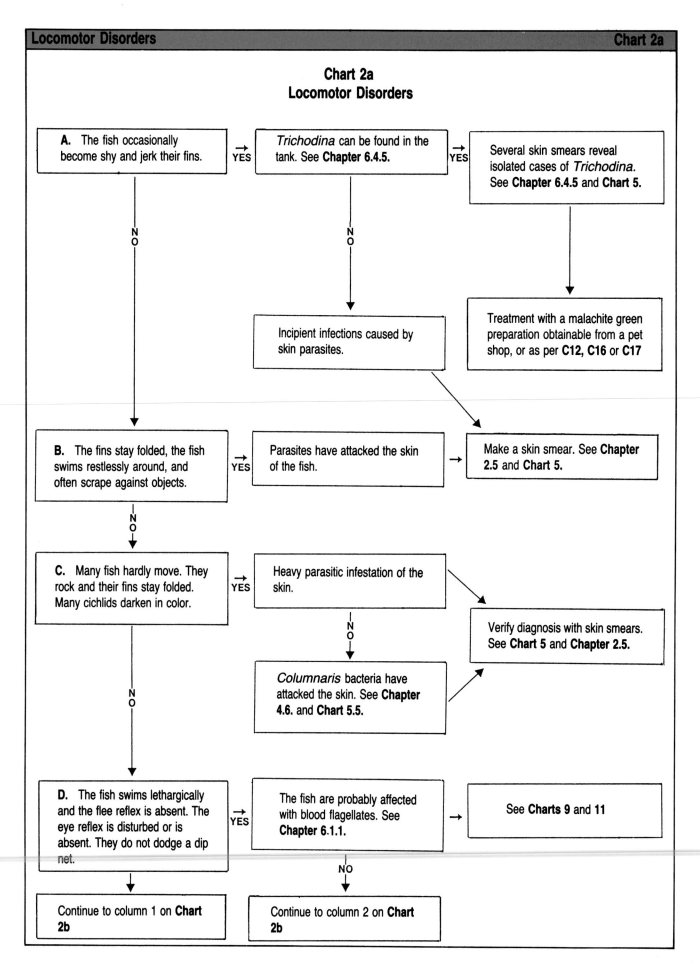

**Chart 2a
Locomotor Disorders**

A. The fish occasionally become shy and jerk their fins. → YES → *Trichodina* can be found in the tank. See **Chapter 6.4.5.** → YES → Several skin smears reveal isolated cases of *Trichodina*. See **Chapter 6.4.5** and **Chart 5.**

NO (from A) ↓

NO (from *Trichodina* box) ↓ Incipient infections caused by skin parasites.

Treatment with a malachite green preparation obtainable from a pet shop, or as per **C12**, **C16** or **C17**

B. The fins stay folded, the fish swims restlessly around, and often scrape against objects. → YES → Parasites have attacked the skin of the fish. → Make a skin smear. See **Chapter 2.5** and **Chart 5.**

NO ↓

C. Many fish hardly move. They rock and their fins stay folded. Many cichlids darken in color. → YES → Heavy parasitic infestation of the skin.

NO ↓ *Columnaris* bacteria have attacked the skin. See **Chapter 4.6.** and **Chart 5.5.**

Verify diagnosis with skin smears. See **Chart 5** and **Chapter 2.5.**

NO ↓

D. The fish swims lethargically and the flee reflex is absent. The eye reflex is disturbed or is absent. They do not dodge a dip net. → YES → The fish are probably affected with blood flagellates. See **Chapter 6.1.1.** → See **Charts 9** and **11**

Continue to column 1 on **Chart 2b**

NO ↓ Continue to column 2 on **Chart 2b**

Chart 2b
Locomotor Disorders (continued)

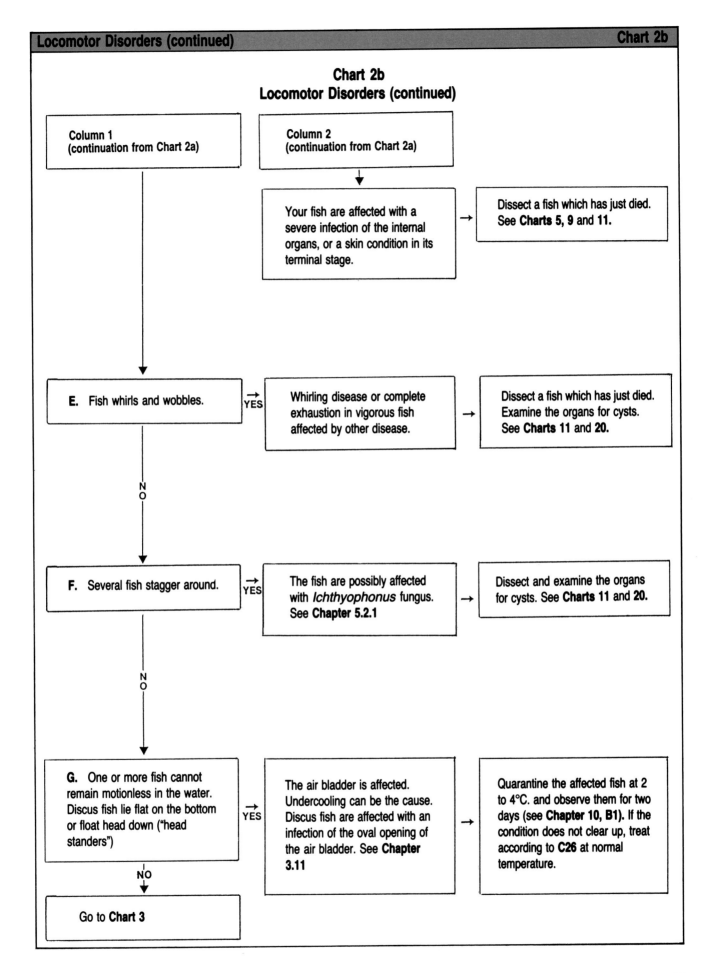

Column 1
(continuation from Chart 2a)

Column 2
(continuation from Chart 2a)

Your fish are affected with a severe infection of the internal organs, or a skin condition in its terminal stage.

→ Dissect a fish which has just died. See **Charts 5, 9** and **11.**

E. Fish whirls and wobbles.

YES → Whirling disease or complete exhaustion in vigorous fish affected by other disease.

→ Dissect a fish which has just died. Examine the organs for cysts. See **Charts 11** and **20.**

NO

F. Several fish stagger around.

YES → The fish are possibly affected with *Ichthyophonus* fungus. See **Chapter 5.2.1**

→ Dissect and examine the organs for cysts. See **Charts 11** and **20.**

NO

G. One or more fish cannot remain motionless in the water. Discus fish lie flat on the bottom or float head down ("head standers")

YES → The air bladder is affected. Undercooling can be the cause. Discus fish are affected with an infection of the oval opening of the air bladder. See **Chapter 3.11**

→ Quarantine the affected fish at 2 to 4°C. and observe them for two days (see **Chapter 10, B1).** If the condition does not clear up, treat according to **C26** at normal temperature.

NO

Go to **Chart 3**

Chart 3a
PHYSICAL CHANGES

A. Do young fish exhibit crippling or deformation? → YES → Considerable damage may be involved. → Fish with hereditary diseases should not be bred. See **Chapter 9.2.**

NO ↓

Developmental anomalies. The fish exhibit shortened, spread out or curled up opercula. Fin anomalies, too, often appear. → Not hereditary. Usually due to deficiencies during development. See **Chapter 9.3.**

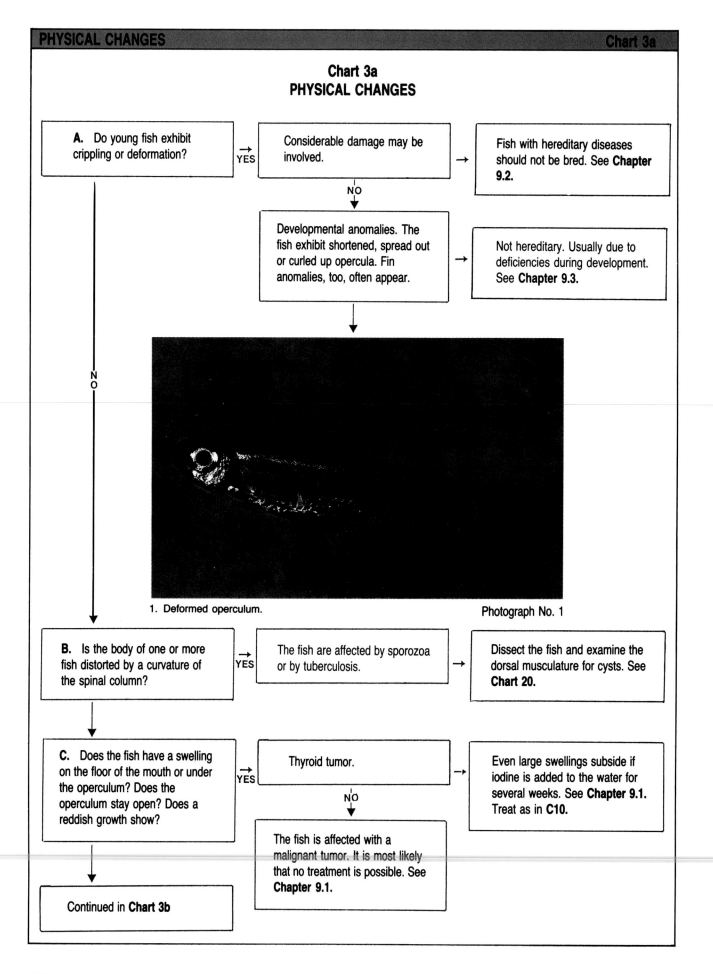

1. Deformed operculum.

Photograph No. 1

B. Is the body of one or more fish distorted by a curvature of the spinal column? → YES → The fish are affected by sporozoa or by tuberculosis. → Dissect the fish and examine the dorsal musculature for cysts. See **Chart 20.**

C. Does the fish have a swelling on the floor of the mouth or under the operculum? Does the operculum stay open? Does a reddish growth show? → YES → Thyroid tumor. → Even large swellings subside if iodine is added to the water for several weeks. See **Chapter 9.1.** Treat as in **C10.**

NO ↓

The fish is affected with a malignant tumor. It is most likely that no treatment is possible. See **Chapter 9.1.**

Continued in **Chart 3b**

Chart 3b
PHYSICAL CHANGES (continued)

Continuation of Chart 3a

D. Do the eyes slowly begin to protrude?

→ YES

The fish is affected by a bacterial infection of the internal organs. Tuberculosis and abdominal dropsy are usually expressed in this manner.

→

Dissect the fish and examine the fluid of the body cavity and the organs for bacteria. See **Chart 11.**

NO

E. One or more fish have swollen bodies.

→ YES

Any of a diversity of diseases can be involved. See **Chart 11.**

NO

F. Many fish lose weight and show a sharp edge to the ridge of the dorsum. The body sinks in, the fish darkens in color. The eyes can also sink in.

→ YES

Your fish probably are affected with intestinal flagellates or worms.

→

Examine a fecal smear under the microscope. See **Chart 8.**

NO

Tuberculosis or abdominal dropsy can also be the cause.

→

Dissect the dead fish. See **Charts 9** and 11.

NO

Continued in **Chart 3c**

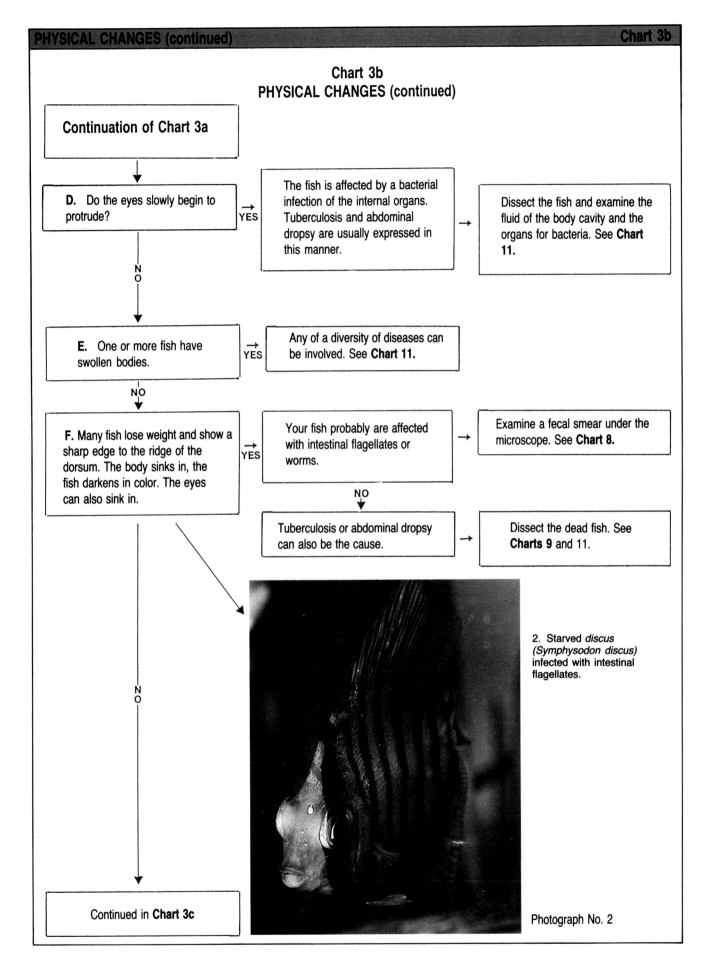

2. Starved *discus* (*Symphysodon discus*) infected with intestinal flagellates.

Photograph No. 2

**Chart 3c
PHYSICAL CHANGES (continued)**

Continuation from Chart 3b

↓ NO

G. The eyes of one or more fish become cloudy.

→ YES → Were the fish just shipped or carried in an plastic bucket? → YES → The cornea is somewhat abraded. It will regenerate within two days. To encourage healing some methylene blue can be added to the water. See **Chapters 10, C17d** and **C1A**

↓ NO

Worm larvae are found in the eye (worm cataract). Examine with a magnifying glass.

→ YES → The disease cannot spread in the aquarium. With preventive measures, the fish can live a long time.

↓ NO

Bacterial infection of the eye. Quarantine the fish and treat according to methods **C17b** and **C1b.** Examination can be continued by smears. See **Chart 5,** then **Chart 21.**

H. The eye does not become cloudy, but is destroyed from within, and caves in, killing the fish.

→ YES → A fungal infection is present. → Treatment according to **C9** is possible, but usually not successful. Immediately quarantine affected fish.

↓ NO

Continued in **Chart 3d**

Photograph No. 3

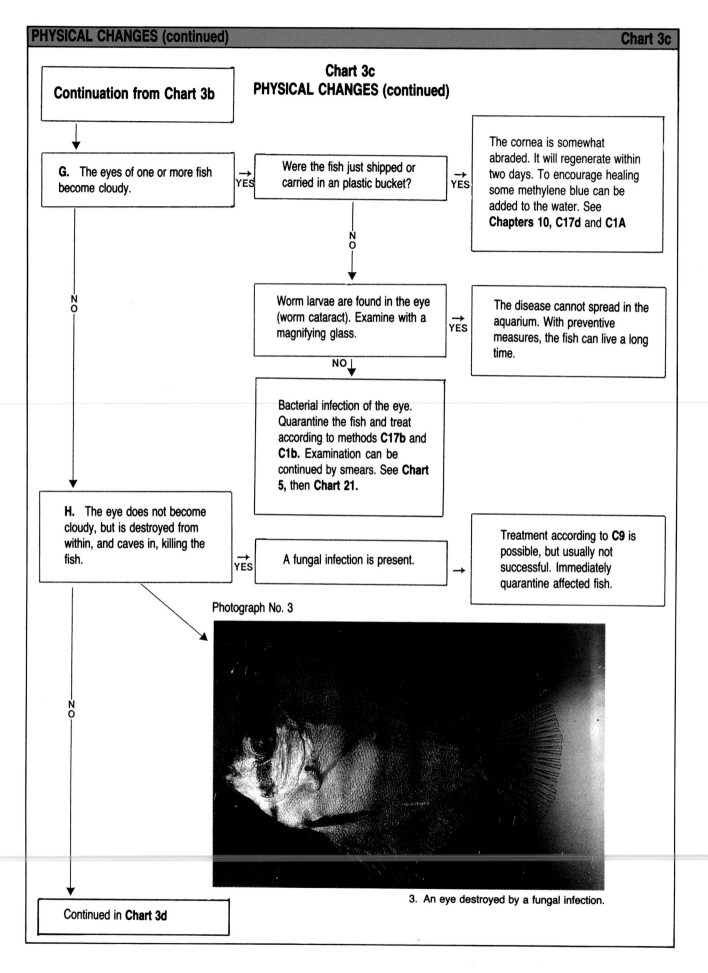

3. An eye destroyed by a fungal infection.

Chart 3d
PHYSICAL CHANGES (continued)

Continuation from Chart 3c

I. Your fish received a wound by fighting with others of its own species, or injured itself on the landscaping objects in the tank! See **Chapter 9.4.**

→ YES

Immediately isolate the fish by transferring it to a quarantine tank. Prevent bacterial or fungal infection of the wound by treating according to **C17d** and **C23.**

NO

K. The fish looks like tiny chunks have been torn out of its body. The wound edges are bloody.

→ YES

The fish has open tuberculosis. Take care! Do not reach into the water if your hands have cuts or other breaks in the skin! See **Chapter 4.7.**

→

Take smears from the wounds and prepare microscope mounts. See **Charts 20** and **21.**

NO

Photograph No. 4

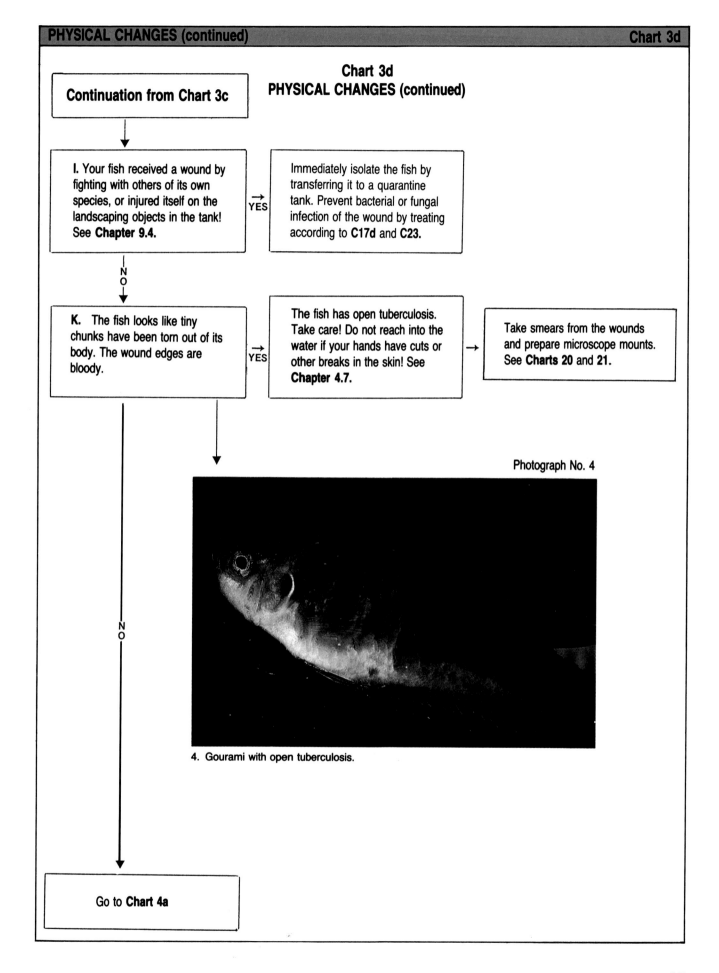

4. Gourami with open tuberculosis.

Go to **Chart 4a**

15

Chart 5a
SKIN

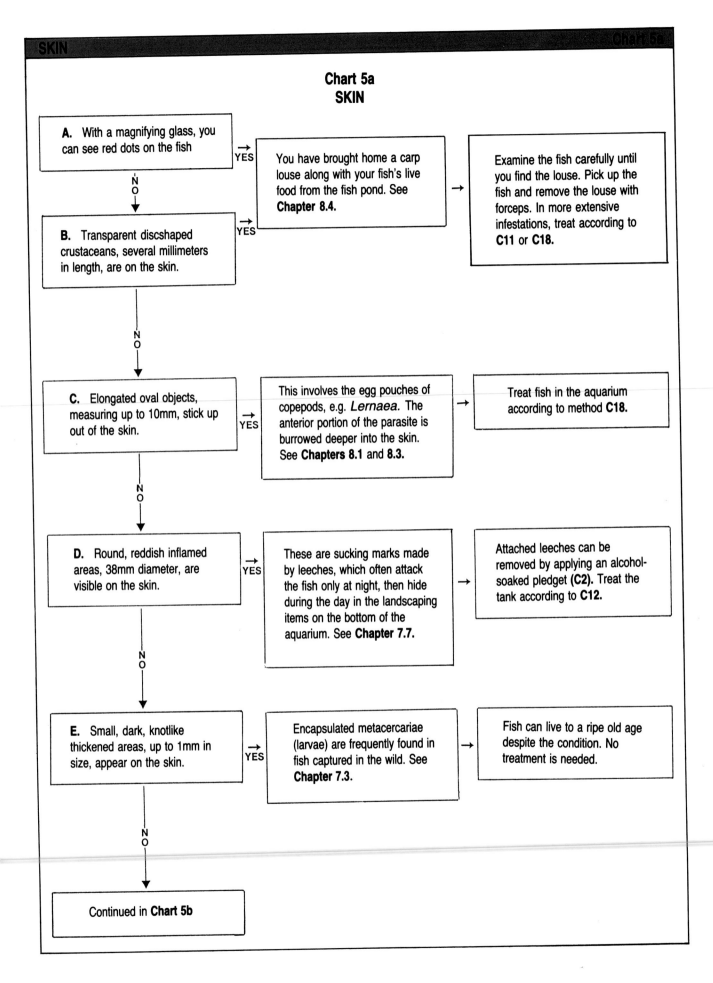

A. With a magnifying glass, you can see red dots on the fish

→ YES → You have brought home a carp louse along with your fish's live food from the fish pond. See **Chapter 8.4.**

→ Examine the fish carefully until you find the louse. Pick up the fish and remove the louse with forceps. In more extensive infestations, treat according to **C11** or **C18.**

NO ↓

B. Transparent discshaped crustaceans, several millimeters in length, are on the skin.

→ YES

NO ↓

C. Elongated oval objects, measuring up to 10mm, stick up out of the skin.

→ YES → This involves the egg pouches of copepods, e.g. *Lernaea.* The anterior portion of the parasite is burrowed deeper into the skin. See **Chapters 8.1** and **8.3.**

→ Treat fish in the aquarium according to method **C18.**

NO ↓

D. Round, reddish inflamed areas, 38mm diameter, are visible on the skin.

→ YES → These are sucking marks made by leeches, which often attack the fish only at night, then hide during the day in the landscaping items on the bottom of the aquarium. See **Chapter 7.7.**

→ Attached leeches can be removed by applying an alcohol-soaked pledget **(C2).** Treat the tank according to **C12.**

NO ↓

E. Small, dark, knotlike thickened areas, up to 1mm in size, appear on the skin.

→ YES → Encapsulated metacercariae (larvae) are frequently found in fish captured in the wild. See **Chapter 7.3.**

→ Fish can live to a ripe old age despite the condition. No treatment is needed.

NO ↓

Continued in **Chart 5b**

Continued from Chart 5a.

Chart 5b
SKIN (continued)

Take smears and begin treatment at once. A delay can be fatal for many fish. Treat according to **C16**.

F. The fish appear to be sprinkled with sand or grit. The lumps are white and have a diameter of 0.5 to 1.5mm. In the terminal stage, the skin comes off in shreds.

→ YES

In the case of freshwater fish, they are affected by the protozoan *Ichthyophthirius*. See **Chapter 6.4.1.**

NO

Marine fish are affected by *Cryptocaryon irritans*. See **Chapter 6.4.2.** size 1-2mm.

→ Choose method **C14** or **C15**. Verify diagnosis by taking a smear.

NO

7. *Ichthyophthirius multifiliis* in a firemouth cichlid, *Cichlasoma meeki.*

G. Isolated white dots, 0.3 to 1mm in size, appear on the skin.

NO

YES

You have discovered an incipient *Ichthyophthirius* infection on your freshwater fish. See **Chapter 6.4.1.**

Treatment can be either according to **B1** or **B2**. The **C16** method is the most rapid.

Photograph No. 7

H. Clearly delineated, whitish, translucent areas measuring 1 to 3mm appear on the skin, often visible only from a head-on view.

8. *Symphysodon discus* infected with *Chilodonella.*

NO

YES

Your fish are affected by the protozoan ciliate *Chilodonella*. See **Chapter 6.4.3.**

A smear often reveals more of the pathogens. Treatment is according to method **C12**, **C17**, **C16** or **C1b.**

Continued in **Chart 5c**

Photograph No. 8

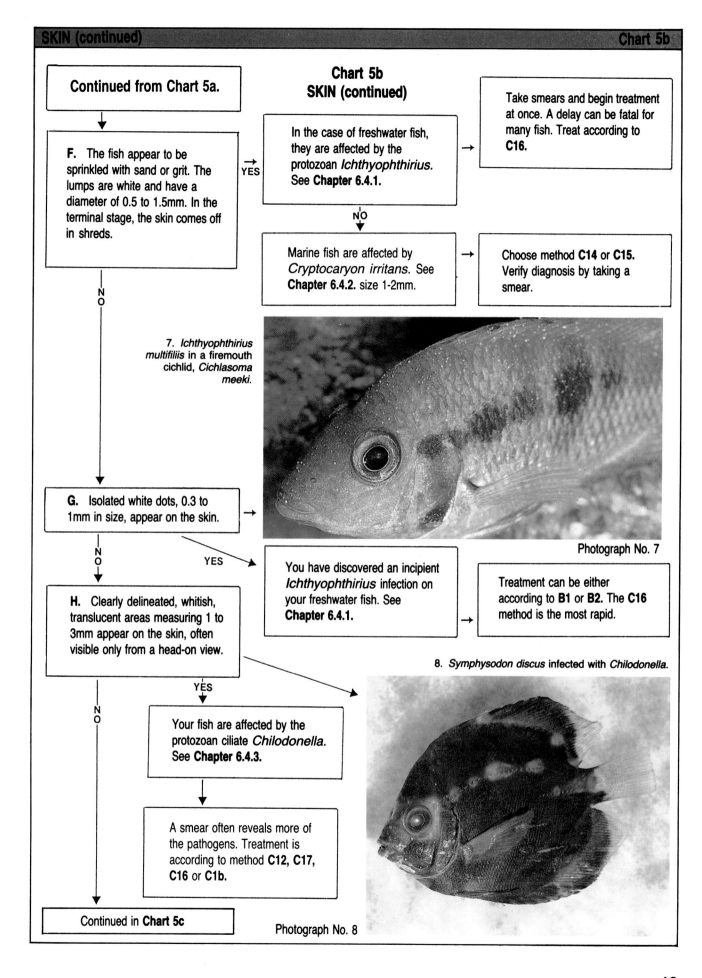

19

Chart 5c
SKIN (continued)

Continued from Chart 5b

↓

I. In marine fish, heavy slime production, along with loss of appetite, lethargy and labored breathing. In the terminal stage, skin slabs come off.

→ YES

Your fish is affected with *Brooklynella hostilis.* See **Chapter 6.4.4.**

→

At the slightest suspicion, immediately take skin and gill smears in order to definitely verify presence of the parasite. Immediately treat according to **C16b** or **C7.**

NO ↓

K. Tiny, dirty-whitish to yellowish dots up to 0.3mm in size appear on the skin and scale edges. (Use a magnifying glass).

→ YES

The fish are affected with *Oodinium,* which can occur in freshwater or marine species. See **Chapter 6.1.3.3.**

→

Take a skin smear and examine under the microscope.

Photograph No. 9

→

N O

↓

L. The skin clouds up in some areas, then comes off, leaving bloody patches.

→ YES

Your fish are affected by an extra heavy *Costia* infection. Bacteria, too, are probably present. See **Chapter 6.1.3.1.**

9. Heavy *Oodinium pillularis* infection, with partial mucosal involvement in *Trichogaster pectoralis.*

→

If possible, increase the temperature to over 30 C, then treat immediately according to **C12, C13** or **C1c.** Examine smears at 400 to 800 X to see *Costia* organisms.

N O

↓

10. *Symphysodon discus* with *Costia* infection. Heavy infection of *Costia* spp, destroying large areas of skin.

Photograph No. 10

M. Whitish, translucent areas not caused by slime form on the skin.

→ YES

The fish are probably affected by sporozoa. See **Chapter 6.3.**

→

Prepare a squash mount from muscle. Many spores will be pressed out from any cysts found there. Method **C22** helps in rare cases. See **Chart 20.**

NO ↓

Continued in **Chart 5d**

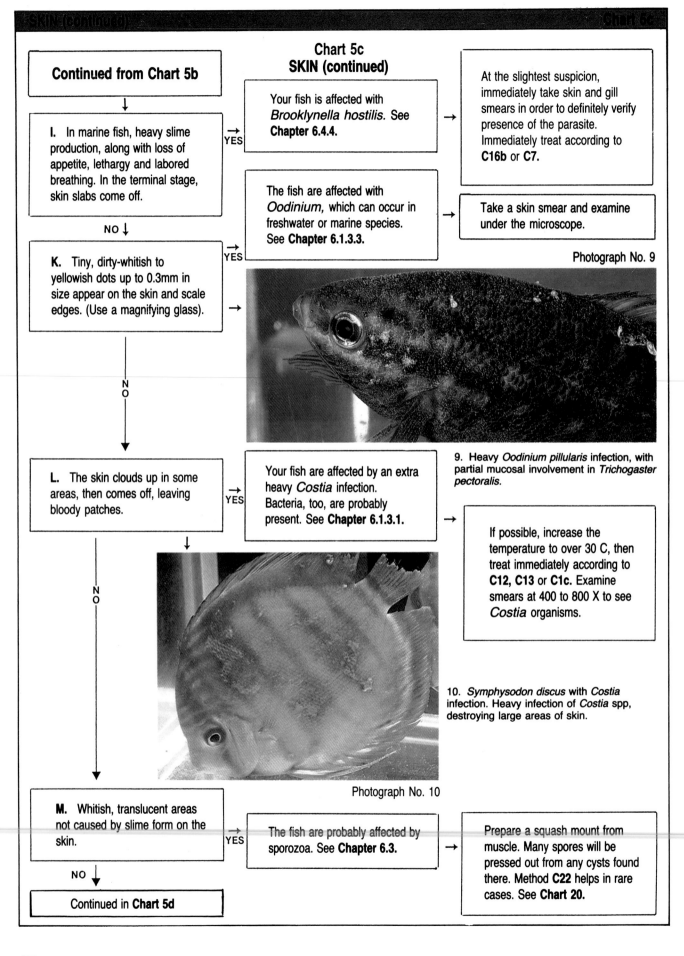

Continued from Chart 5c.

Chart 5d
SKIN (continued)

N. In neons, the color band is interrupted, and the musculature, cloudy and white, shows through.

→ YES

The fish are affected by the sporozoan Plistophora. See **Chapter 6.3.3.1**

→

Treatment is not possible, and the fish should be sacrificed. See **Chart 20.**

NO

O. The skin becomes cloudy. In neons, the color band at this spot looks pale.

→ YES

Is the pH too high?

→ YES

Determine cause. Lower pH by changing the water. See **Chapter 9.5.2.**

NO

The skin is attacked by parasites or bacteria. Take a smear.

NO

P. The skin, cloudy and inflamed in places, produces a great deal of slime.

→ YES

Does the pH satisfy the needs of the fish?

→ YES

The skin is heavily infected with either parasites or bacteria.

NO

Extreme fluctuations in pH, too, lead to slime production in the skin. Adjust pH by changing the water. See **Chapter 9.5.2.**

Rapid countermeasures are required. Quarantine the fish and treat according to **C12, C176, C13, C9** or **C23.**

NO

Q. White threads grow out of white-and-red-edged wounds, and form cottony puffs.

→ YES

Fungus is infecting the wound. See **Chapter 5.1.**

→

11. Skin sites attacked by fungus following injury.

Photograph No. 11

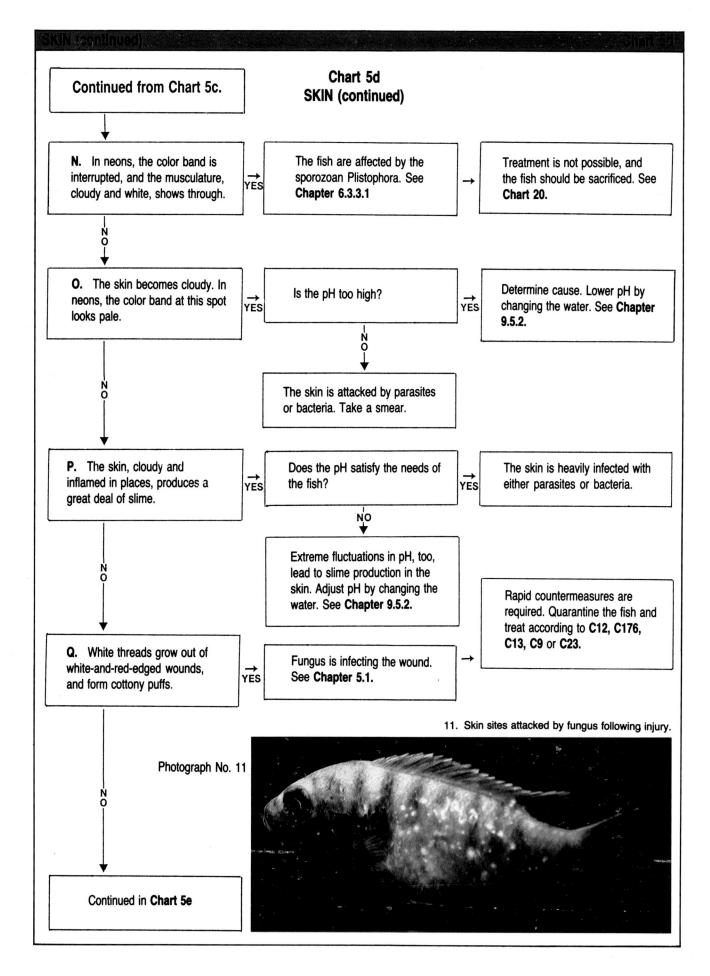

NO

Continued in **Chart 5e**

Continued from Chart 5d

Chart 5e
SKIN (continued)

R. A whitish film forms around the mouth on one or more fish.

→ YES

This is a bacterial infection presumably *Columnaris* of the skin. See **Chapters 4.4** and **4.6.**

→

Definitive diagnosis can only be made by microscopic examination of a smear. See **Chart 21.**

NO

Photograph No. 12

12. White spots on skin and scale margins in a *Columnaris* infection.

S. The scales in many places are outlined in white. The skin easily becomes slimy. The fish folds its fins and sways.

→

→ YES

The skin is heavily invaded by *Columnaris* bacteria. See **Chapter 4.6.**

→

Verify diagnosis by smear. **See Chart 21.**

NO

T. Redbordered lesions in the skin. They often clear up spontaneously.

→ YES

The lesions rupture, releasing a purulent liquid.

→ YES

Bacteria cause the lesions. Mount a specimen of the purulent liquid and examine under the microscope. See **Chapter 4.3.** See also **Charts 20** and **21.**

NO

Lesions rupture, but nothing is released.

→ YES

The fish is affected with open tuberculosis. See **Chapter 4.7.** No treatment is possible, and the fish should be sacrificed.

NO

13. Rainbow fish with tuberculosis.

Photograph 13

Continued in Chart 5f

Extract some of the lesion's contents and stain with Ziehl-Neelsen. See **Chapter 11.8.7.** See also **Charts 20** and **21.**

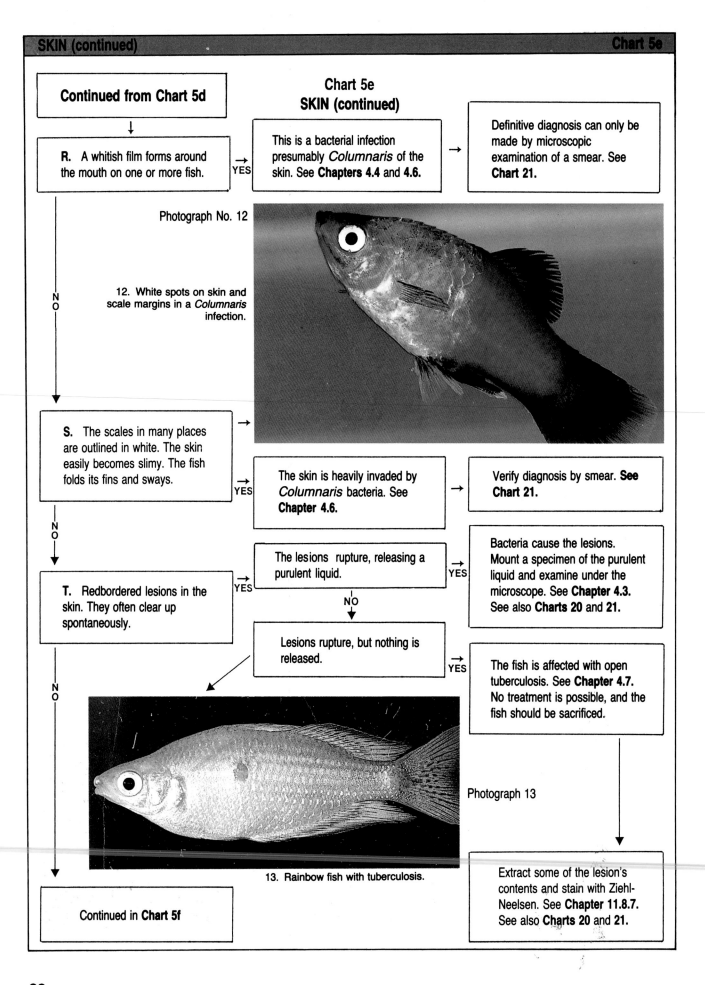

Chart 5f
SKIN (concluded)

Continued from Chart 5e

↓

U. A swelling forms in the muscle under the skin during the course of several weeks, and may protrude way out from the surface of the body. The scales can be lifted, too, at the site.

→ YES → A sporozoan cyst or lesion forms in the musculature. See **Chapters 6.3** and **9.1.**

→ Open the lesion and prepare a mount to examine for diagnosis. See **Chart 20.**

NO ↓

We are dealing with a case of bloat here.

The fish is affected with abdominal dropsy. See also **Chart 3 (parts D and E).**

→ Verify the diagnosis by dissection. See **Chart 11.**

N O ↓

V. Blisters form along the lateral line. Often associated with bloat, spread scales and popeyes.

→ YES

N O ↓

Photograph No.

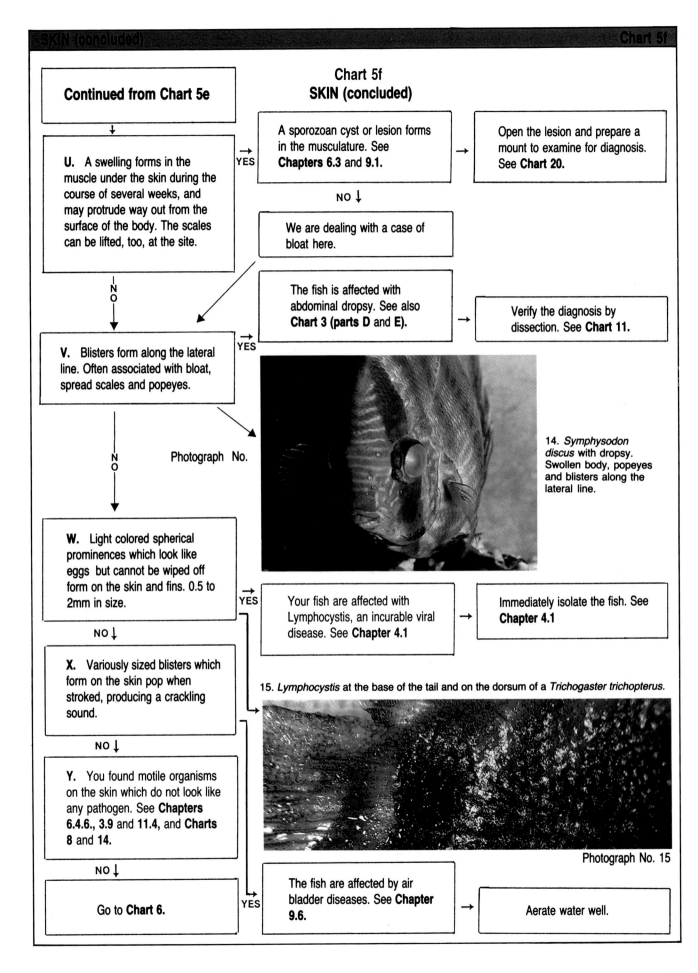

14. *Symphysodon discus* with dropsy. Swollen body, popeyes and blisters along the lateral line.

W. Light colored spherical prominences which look like eggs but cannot be wiped off form on the skin and fins. 0.5 to 2mm in size.

→ YES → Your fish are affected with Lymphocystis, an incurable viral disease. See **Chapter 4.1**

→ Immediately isolate the fish. See **Chapter 4.1**

NO ↓

X. Variously sized blisters which form on the skin pop when stroked, producing a crackling sound.

15. *Lymphocystis* at the base of the tail and on the dorsum of a *Trichogaster trichopterus.*

NO ↓

Y. You found motile organisms on the skin which do not look like any pathogen. See **Chapters 6.4.6., 3.9** and **11.4,** and **Charts 8** and **14.**

Photograph No. 15

NO ↓

Go to **Chart 6.**

→ YES → The fish are affected by air bladder diseases. See **Chapter 9.6.**

→ Aerate water well.

Chart 6a
FINS

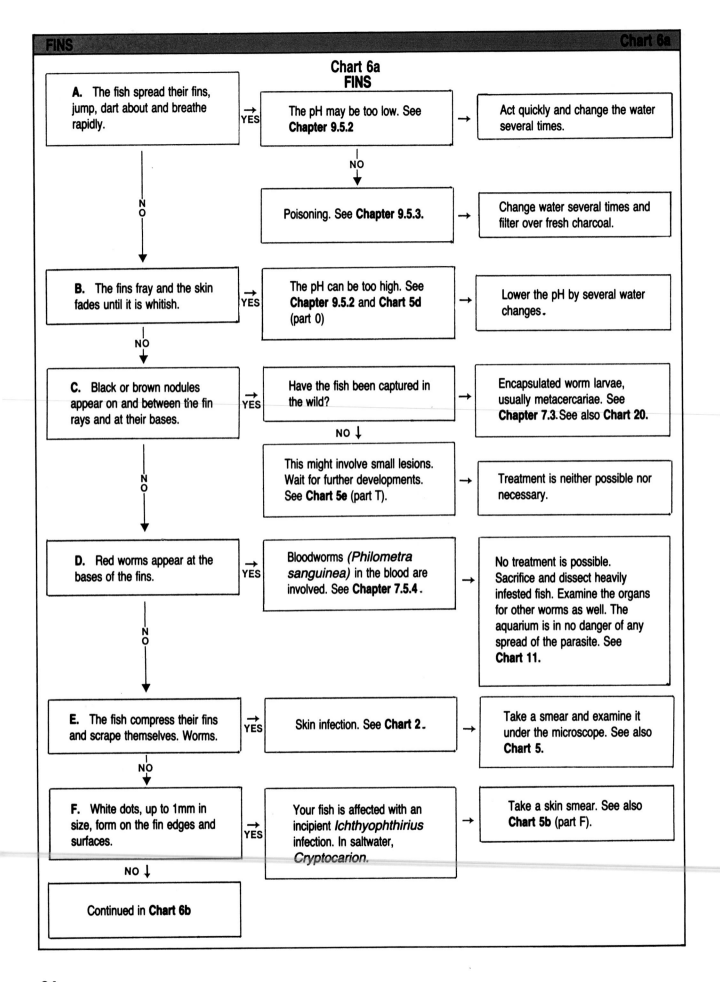

A. The fish spread their fins, jump, dart about and breathe rapidly.

→ YES → The pH may be too low. See **Chapter 9.5.2** → Act quickly and change the water several times.

NO ↓

Poisoning. See **Chapter 9.5.3.** → Change water several times and filter over fresh charcoal.

NO ↓

B. The fins fray and the skin fades until it is whitish.

→ YES → The pH can be too high. See **Chapter 9.5.2** and **Chart 5d** (part 0) → Lower the pH by several water changes.

NO ↓

C. Black or brown nodules appear on and between the fin rays and at their bases.

→ YES → Have the fish been captured in the wild? → Encapsulated worm larvae, usually metacercariae. See **Chapter 7.3.** See also **Chart 20.**

NO ↓

This might involve small lesions. Wait for further developments. See **Chart 5e** (part T). → Treatment is neither possible nor necessary.

NO ↓

D. Red worms appear at the bases of the fins.

→ YES → Bloodworms *(Philometra sanguinea)* in the blood are involved. See **Chapter 7.5.4.** → No treatment is possible. Sacrifice and dissect heavily infested fish. Examine the organs for other worms as well. The aquarium is in no danger of any spread of the parasite. See **Chart 11.**

NO ↓

E. The fish compress their fins and scrape themselves. Worms.

→ YES → Skin infection. See **Chart 2.** → Take a smear and examine it under the microscope. See also **Chart 5.**

NO ↓

F. White dots, up to 1mm in size, form on the fin edges and surfaces.

→ YES → Your fish is affected with an incipient *Ichthyophthirius* infection. In saltwater, *Cryptocarion.* → Take a skin smear. See also **Chart 5b** (part F).

NO ↓

Continued in **Chart 6b**

Chart 6b
FINS

Continued from Chart 6a

NO ↓

G. A velvety coating forms on the fin edges and the sides. With a hand lens, the individual dots are visible.

→ YES

Your fish are affected with *Oodinium*.

→

Take a smear. **See Chart 5c** (part K).

NO ↓

H. The fins, edged in white, grow shorter and shorter.

→ YES

Bacterial fin rot (see **Chapter 4.4**) or too high a pH. See **Chart 6a** (part B).

→

Improve water quality. Take a smear. See **Chart 5.**

16. Bacterial fin rot on the tail (i.e., tail rot).

Photograph No. 16

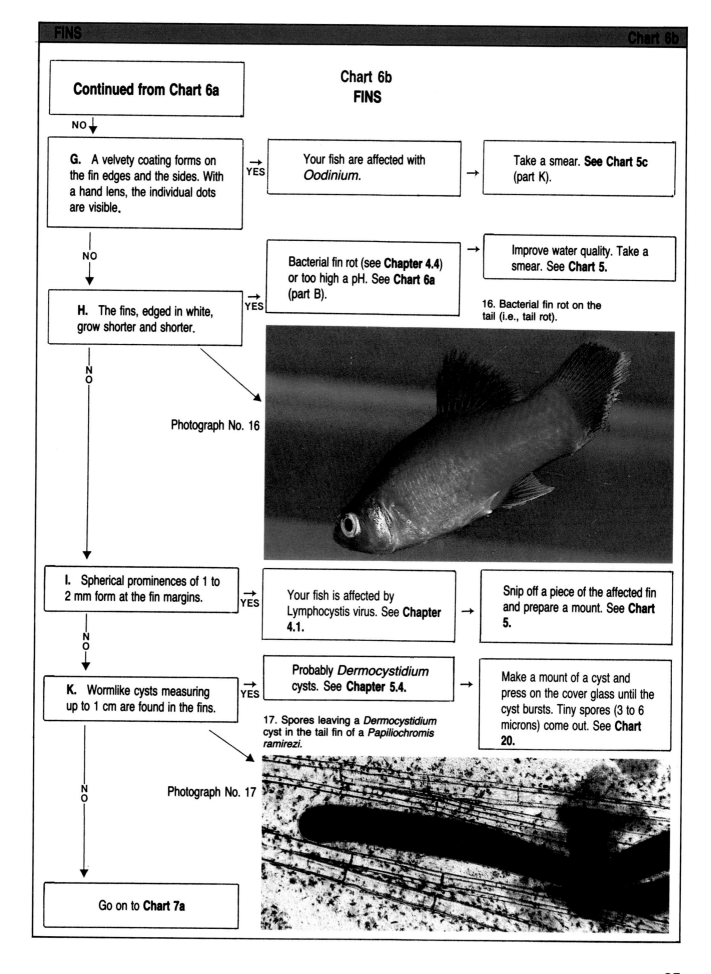

NO ↓

I. Spherical prominences of 1 to 2 mm form at the fin margins.

→ YES

Your fish is affected by Lymphocystis virus. See **Chapter 4.1.**

→

Snip off a piece of the affected fin and prepare a mount. See **Chart 5.**

NO ↓

K. Wormlike cysts measuring up to 1 cm are found in the fins.

→ YES

Probably *Dermocystidium* cysts. See **Chapter 5.4.**

→

Make a mount of a cyst and press on the cover glass until the cyst bursts. Tiny spores (3 to 6 microns) come out. See **Chart 20.**

17. Spores leaving a *Dermocystidium* cyst in the tail fin of a *Papiliochromis ramirezi.*

Photograph No. 17

NO ↓

Go on to **Chart 7a**

25

Chart 7a
GILLS

You should first read **Chapters 2** and **3** to be able to carry out the following examinations.

A. The gill filaments are light, having lost color.

→ YES

Has the pH changed? Is chlorine in the water? Is ammonia in the water? See **Chapter 9.5.** See also **Chart 6a** (parts A and B) and **Chart 1**

→ YES

Establish optimal water values!

NO ↓

The fish can be affected by a kidney disease. See further below under M.

NO ↓

B. Small, white objects (1 to 1.5mm) are attached to the gill filaments. They hold very tightly.

→ YES

Gill crustaceans. See **Chapter 8.2**

→

With pointed forceps or tweezers, pick off a few specimens and examine them under the microscope. Treat according to **C18, C11** or **C7.**

NO ↓

C. Blood-red worms are visible on the inside surface of the operculum, but usually only in pond fish.

→ YES

The fish are affected with bloodworms *(Philometra* spp) See also **Chart 6a** (part D) and **Chapter 7.5.4.**

→

No treatment possible. Dissect the fish and examine the organs. See **Charts 9** and **11.**

NO ↓

D. Light flecks appear on the gills. The gill filaments are necrotic at these spots.

→ YES

With finely pointed forceps, remove some of these dead filaments and examine at 100X. Does the mount contain extremely flattened dropletshaped eggs?

→ YES

Eggs of the blood fluke *Sanguinicola* spp are involved. See **Chapter 7.3**

NO ↓

Continued in **Chart 7b**

NO ↓

If fungal hyphae are seen in the mount, then gill rot is involved.

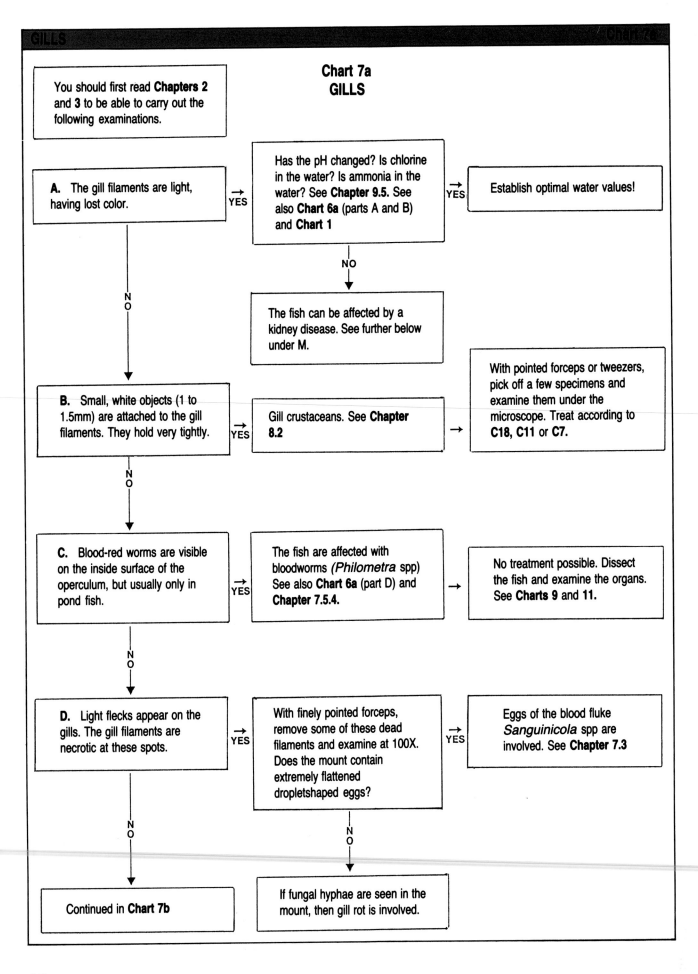

Continued from Chart 7a

**Chart 7b
GILLS (continued)**

E. Are the gills flecked with gray-white? Do the filaments keep on falling out?

→ YES

Branchiomyces fungal gill rot. See **Chapter 5.2.3.**

→

Confirm the diagnosis by preparing a mount. Treat according to **C12, C17b, C9** or **C3. See also Chart 10** (part C).

Photograph No. 18

NO

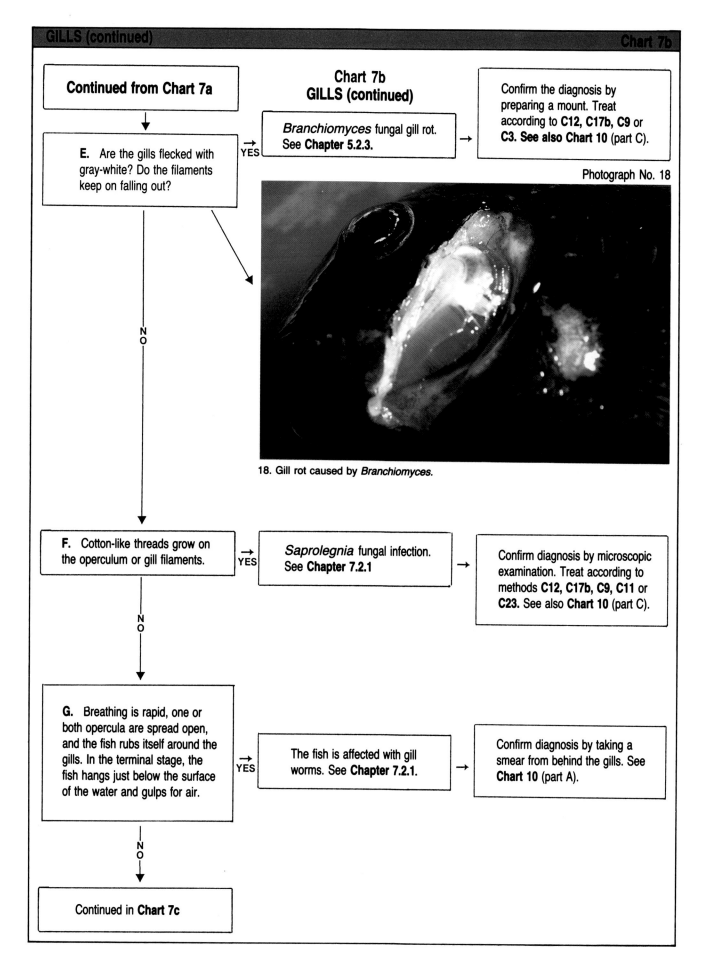

18. Gill rot caused by *Branchiomyces*.

F. Cotton-like threads grow on the operculum or gill filaments.

→ YES

Saprolegnia fungal infection. See **Chapter 7.2.1**

→

Confirm diagnosis by microscopic examination. Treat according to methods **C12, C17b, C9, C11** or **C23. See also Chart 10** (part C).

NO

G. Breathing is rapid, one or both opercula are spread open, and the fish rubs itself around the gills. In the terminal stage, the fish hangs just below the surface of the water and gulps for air.

→ YES

The fish is affected with gill worms. See **Chapter 7.2.1.**

→

Confirm diagnosis by taking a smear from behind the gills. See **Chart 10** (part A).

NO

Continued in **Chart 7c**

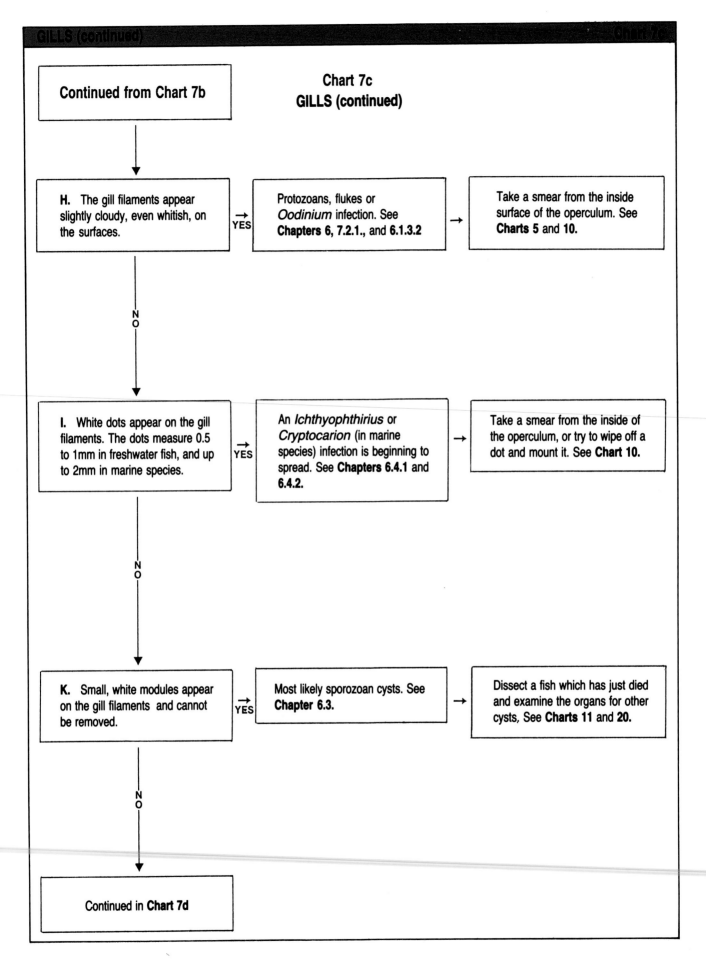

Continued from Chart 7b

Chart 7c
GILLS (continued)

H. The gill filaments appear slightly cloudy, even whitish, on the surfaces.

→ YES → Protozoans, flukes or *Oodinium* infection. See **Chapters 6, 7.2.1.,** and **6.1.3.2**

→ Take a smear from the inside surface of the operculum. See **Charts 5** and **10.**

NO

I. White dots appear on the gill filaments. The dots measure 0.5 to 1mm in freshwater fish, and up to 2mm in marine species.

→ YES → An *Ichthyophthirius* or *Cryptocarion* (in marine species) infection is beginning to spread. See **Chapters 6.4.1** and **6.4.2.**

→ Take a smear from the inside of the operculum, or try to wipe off a dot and mount it. See **Chart 10.**

NO

K. Small, white modules appear on the gill filaments and cannot be removed.

→ YES → Most likely sporozoan cysts. See **Chapter 6.3.**

→ Dissect a fish which has just died and examine the organs for other cysts, See **Charts 11** and **20.**

NO

Continued in **Chart 7d**

Chart 7d
GILLS (concluded)

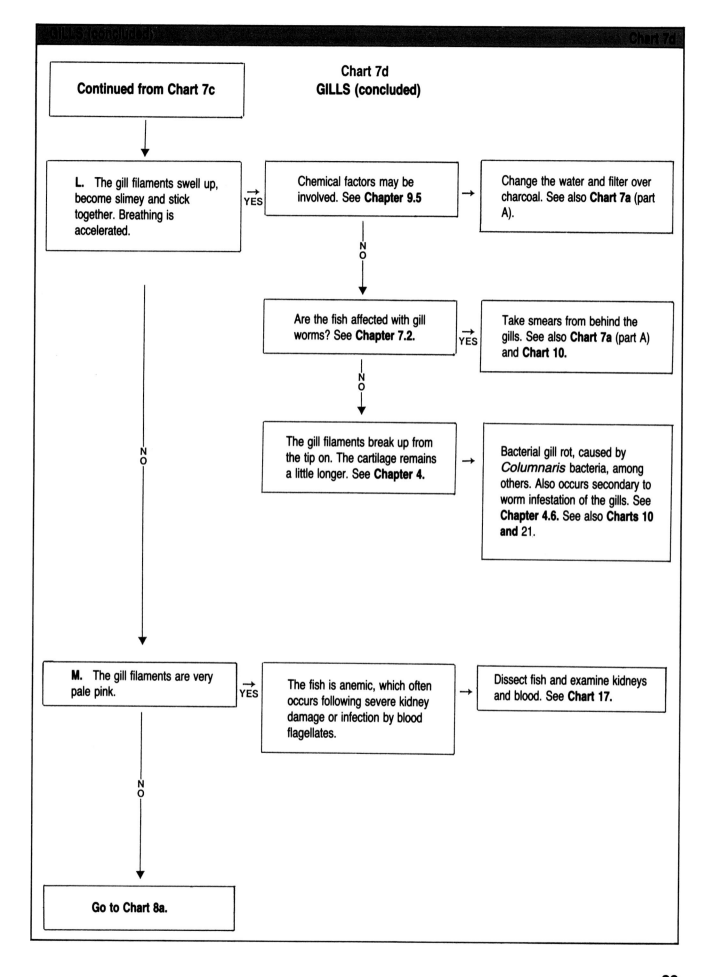

Continued from Chart 7c

L. The gill filaments swell up, become slimey and stick together. Breathing is accelerated.

YES → Chemical factors may be involved. See **Chapter 9.5**

→ Change the water and filter over charcoal. See also **Chart 7a** (part A).

NO ↓

Are the fish affected with gill worms? See **Chapter 7.2.**

YES → Take smears from behind the gills. See also **Chart 7a** (part A) and **Chart 10.**

NO ↓

The gill filaments break up from the tip on. The cartilage remains a little longer. See **Chapter 4.**

→ Bacterial gill rot, caused by *Columnaris* bacteria, among others. Also occurs secondary to worm infestation of the gills. See **Chapter 4.6.** See also **Charts 10 and** 21.

NO ↓

M. The gill filaments are very pale pink.

YES → The fish is anemic, which often occurs following severe kidney damage or infection by blood flagellates.

→ Dissect fish and examine kidneys and blood. See **Chart 17.**

NO ↓

Go to Chart 8a.

29

A. The vent or anal area is inflamed, and feces are often slimey.

Chart 8a
FECES

YES →

The rectum is inflamed.

→ Carefully take a smear of material at the anus. Try to express a tiny amount of feces by gently applying some pressure. Prepare a smear. See Part E in **Chart 8b.**

N O ↓

B. The vent does not appear to be inflamed, but no fecal matter can be expressed completely, and is dragged around a while as a long, often slimey thread.

YES →

The intestines are affected. Bacteria, flagellates and/or worms can be the cause.

→ Prepare a fresh fecal mount. See part E in **Chart 8b.**

N O ↓

C. Fecal droppings are white or yellow, and slimey. The fish becomes skinnier.

YES →

Your fish is probably affected with intestinal flagellates. Nematodes can be a secondary cause.

→ Confirm the diagnosis by microscopic examination of a fecal sample not older than 5 minutes. See part E in **Chart 8b.**

N O ↓

The rectum is infected by *Camallanus* worms, which bear live larvae.

→ Do not yank the worms out of the anus with the forceps, or the instestine will be damaged. Treat according to **B3, C5, C6** and **18a.** See also part D in **Chart 14a.**

D. When the fish remain stationary, red or brown worms hang about 5 to 10 mm out of the anus, which is dilated.

YES →

→

Photograph No. 19

19. *Camallanus cotti* hanging out of the vent of a fish.

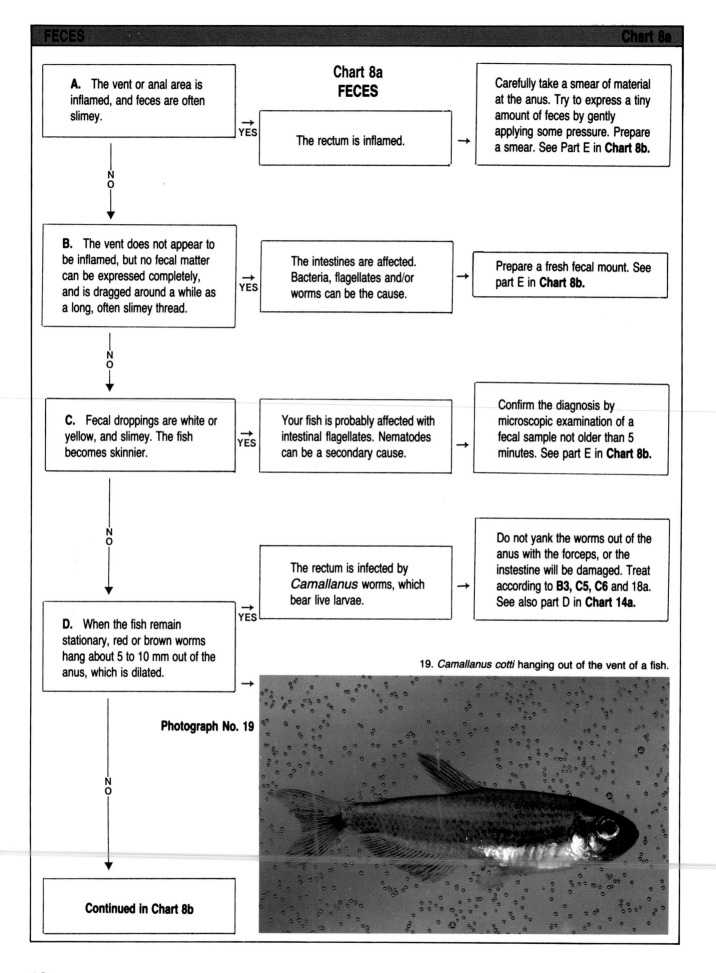

N O ↓

Continued in Chart 8b

Continued from Chart 8a.

Chart 8b
FECES (continued)

You have prepared a fecal mount and are now examining it under the microscope at 50 to 100 X. The procedure is described in **Chapter 4.**

E. The feces contain small, thin worms, ranging in size from 1 mm to much smaller.

YES →

This involves the larvae of livebearing nematodes. See **Chapter 7.5.3.**

→

Treatment is according to **B3, C5, C6** or **C18a. See part D of Chart 8a and part D of Chart 14a.**

NO ↓

F. The mounted specimen contains whitish, elongated, flat segments with almost squared-off corners and an intricate inner structure. Several segments often hang together in a chain.

YES →

Your fish has a tapeworm. This usually happens only in fish captured in the wild or from fish farms. See **Chapter 7.4** and **Photograph No. 96.**

→

Control is possible only by feeding medicated food (**C24**) Treatment is not absolutely necessary if the fish are healthy and act normally. See part B **Chart 14.**

NO ↓

G. The feces contain numerous spindle-shaped eggs with pointed ends. Many species have long white threads at the ends.

YES →

The eggs are from thorny-headed worms, usually only in fish from open air sources. The fish are infected via isopods or water fleas, which carry the larvae of the thorny-headed worms. See Chapter 7.6.

→

Start treatment soon, for the worms damage the intestines. Treatment is according to **C24.** Deep-freeze water fleas (which you plan to use as food) for three days before feeding fish with them. See part A in **Chart 14a.**

NO ↓

H. The feces contain elongated eggs with champagne-cork-like covers. 200 to 400 X.

YES →

The fish harbors one or more *Capillaria* worms. See **Chapter 7.5.1.**

→

The worms reproduce slowly. Treatment is according to **C6** or **C5** in feed **B5.** See part G in **Chart 14b.**

NO ↓

Photograph No. 20

20. *Capillaria* eggs in droppings, size 50-60u.

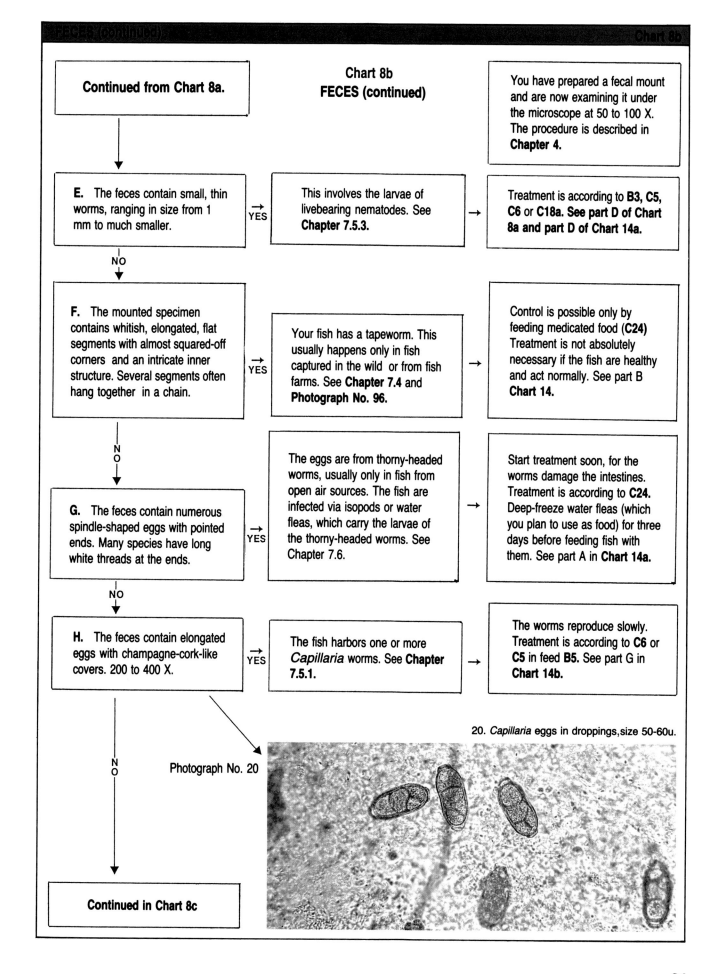

Continued in Chart 8c

Chart 9
Blood

The following examinations are done on a fish which has just died. You should already have read **Chapters 2, 3** and **11**. Proceed as indicated by the dissection guidelines in **Chapter 3.** To do a blood examination by itself, proceed as in **Chapter 3.3.** To proceed most thoroughly, review **Charts 5** and **6** first. Use a sharp scalpel to scrape off skin and snip off fin fragments to prepare mounts.

A. In the blood smear, among the blood cells, you will observe rapidly motile protozoans which measure 14 to 24u.

→ YES

The fish are affected with "fish sleeping sickness," caused by the flagellate *Cryptobia*. See **Chapter 6.1.1.**

→

Treatment can be attempted, but success is uncertain. Treatment is according to method **C17b.**

NO ↓

B. Encapsulated inclusion bodies are seen in the red blood cells.

→ YES

Sporozoans which attack blood cells. Very rare. See **Chapter 6.3.**

→

Treatment is not possible.

NO ↓

C. Bacteria are among and on the blood cells.

→ YES

This can occur in various bacterial diseases. See **Chapter 4.**

→

Close examination of the organs is necessary. See **Chart 21.**

NO ↓

D. The blood cells are deformed or have burst.

→ YES

You made an error in your histological technique! Use physiological saline for preparing the slide. See **Chapter 10** and method **C12.**

NO ↓

Go to Chart 10

Mount dissected gill filaments. The blood from them can be examined as per **Chart 9.**

Chart 10
Gill Filaments

Quick treatment is needed for young fish. They can be treated with Gyrotox or according to methods **C6, C18, C11** or **C7.** In discus fish, only treatment **C18** or **C6** helps.

A. Worms with posterior hooking organs use them to hang on tightly to the gill filaments while probing about with the anterior end of the body.

YES → The gills are attacked by flukes. See **Chapter 7.2.** →

NO

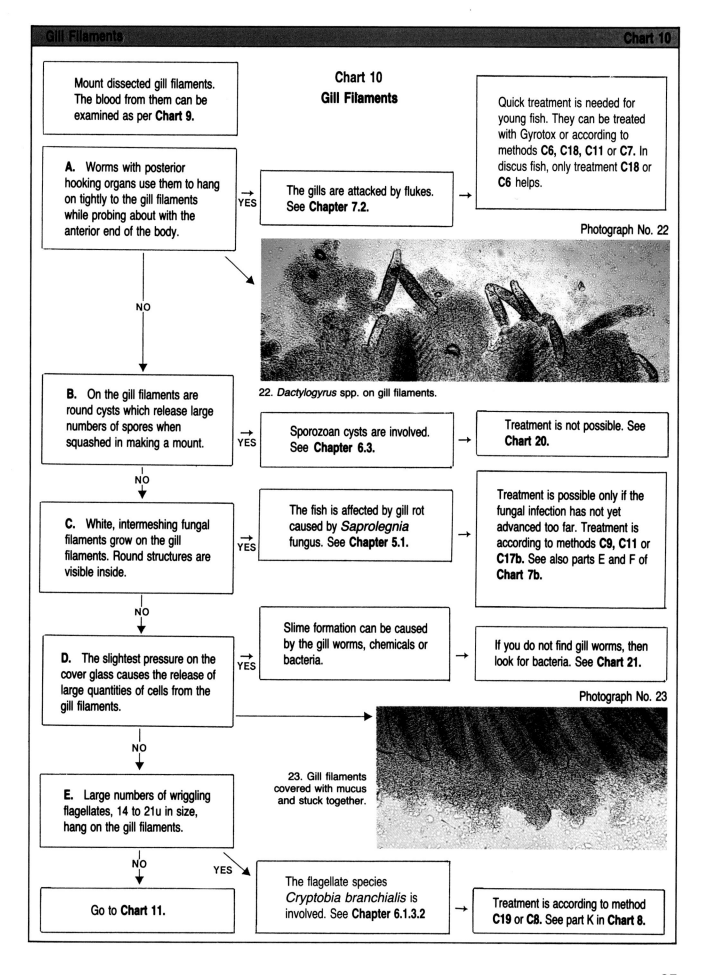

Photograph No. 22

22. *Dactylogyrus* spp. on gill filaments.

B. On the gill filaments are round cysts which release large numbers of spores when squashed in making a mount.

YES → Sporozoan cysts are involved. See **Chapter 6.3.** → Treatment is not possible. See **Chart 20.**

NO

C. White, intermeshing fungal filaments grow on the gill filaments. Round structures are visible inside.

YES → The fish is affected by gill rot caused by *Saprolegnia* fungus. See **Chapter 5.1.** → Treatment is possible only if the fungal infection has not yet advanced too far. Treatment is according to methods **C9, C11** or **C17b.** See also parts E and F of **Chart 7b.**

NO

D. The slightest pressure on the cover glass causes the release of large quantities of cells from the gill filaments.

YES → Slime formation can be caused by the gill worms, chemicals or bacteria. → If you do not find gill worms, then look for bacteria. See **Chart 21.**

NO

Photograph No. 23

23. Gill filaments covered with mucus and stuck together.

E. Large numbers of wriggling flagellates, 14 to 21u in size, hang on the gill filaments.

YES → The flagellate species *Cryptobia branchialis* is involved. See **Chapter 6.1.3.2** → Treatment is according to method **C19** or **C8.** See part K in **Chart 8.**

NO

Go to **Chart 11.**

35

Chart 11a
Body Cavity

A. The body cavity is filled with fluid, which often simply runs out when the abdominal wall is cut open.

→ YES

The fish is affected with abdominal dropsy. See **Chapter 4.2.**

→

Prepare a mount of the fluid and examine for blood and bacteria. Treatment can be according to method **C25, A5, A6** or **A1**. See **Chart 21.**

NO

↓

B. The fluid in the body cavity is viscous, the organs are atrophied and the intestine is glassy.

→ YES

Abdominal dropsy is the problem here, too. See **Chapter 4.2.**

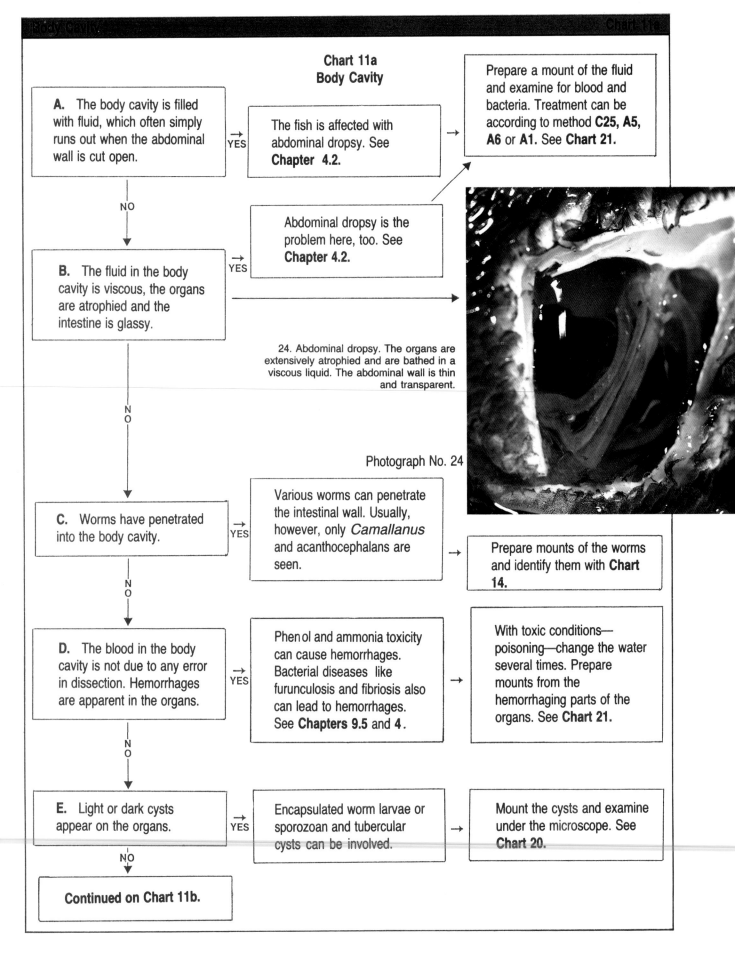

24. Abdominal dropsy. The organs are extensively atrophied and are bathed in a viscous liquid. The abdominal wall is thin and transparent.

Photograph No. 24

NO

↓

C. Worms have penetrated into the body cavity.

→ YES

Various worms can penetrate the intestinal wall. Usually, however, only *Camallanus* and acanthocephalans are seen.

→

Prepare mounts of the worms and identify them with **Chart 14.**

NO

↓

D. The blood in the body cavity is not due to any error in dissection. Hemorrhages are apparent in the organs.

→ YES

Phenol and ammonia toxicity can cause hemorrhages. Bacterial diseases like furunculosis and fibriosis also can lead to hemorrhages. See **Chapters 9.5** and **4**.

→

With toxic conditions— poisoning—change the water several times. Prepare mounts from the hemorrhaging parts of the organs. See **Chart 21.**

NO

↓

E. Light or dark cysts appear on the organs.

→ YES

Encapsulated worm larvae or sporozoan and tubercular cysts can be involved.

→

Mount the cysts and examine under the microscope. See **Chart 20.**

NO

↓

Continued on Chart 11b.

Chart 11b
Body Cavity (concluded)

Continued from Chart 11a.

↓ NO

F. After the side of the body is lifted up, you can see how the turgid anterior gut has displaced the liver to the side.

→ YES

The fish had an intestinal obstruction. You can recognize the undigested food in the intestine. See **Chapter 9.3.**

→

Do other fish have swollen bodies? Raise the temperature by 3 to 5°C. and feed with varied ballast-rich and vitamin-rich food. And, above all, do not give any cold food.

Photograph No. 25

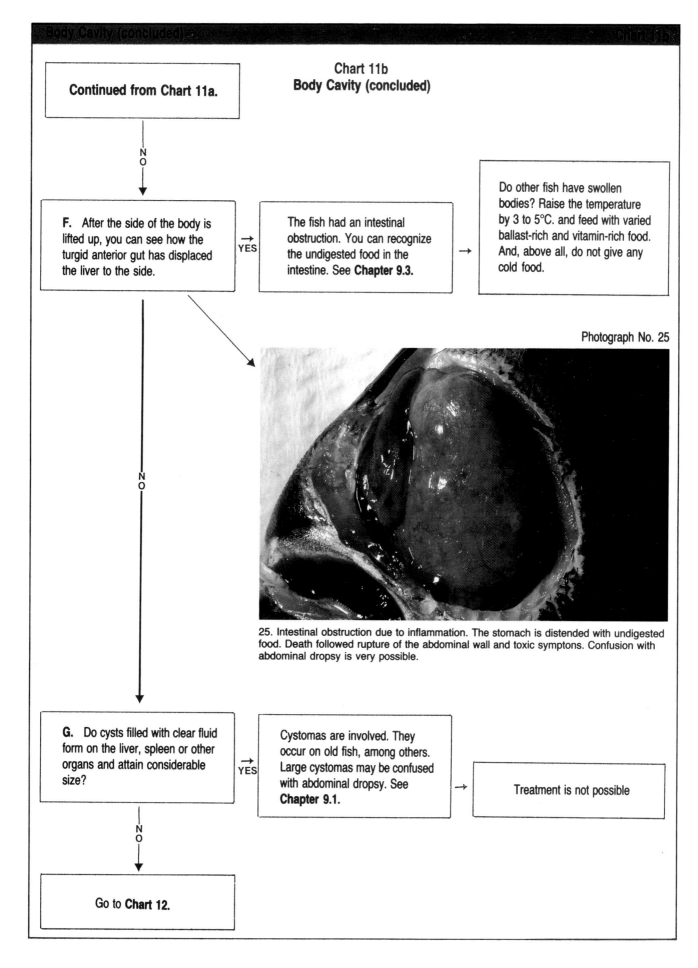

25. Intestinal obstruction due to inflammation. The stomach is distended with undigested food. Death followed rupture of the abdominal wall and toxic symptons. Confusion with abdominal dropsy is very possible.

↓ NO

G. Do cysts filled with clear fluid form on the liver, spleen or other organs and attain considerable size?

→ YES

Cystomas are involved. They occur on old fish, among others. Large cystomas may be confused with abdominal dropsy. See **Chapter 9.1.**

→

Treatment is not possible

↓ NO

Go to **Chart 12.**

Chart 12
Liver

The liver, gallbladder, intestines and spleen are usually removed together. Organs which are not immediately processed should be kept in a small dish filled with physiological saline. Photographs 45 to 47 show what a healthy liver should look like.

A. The liver is discolored brown or yellow. The mounted specimen reveals numerous light-colored fat droplets with dark borders. See Photograph No. 48. → YES →

The cause can be abdominal dropsy or fatty degeneration of the liver due to faulty nutrition or to bacterial infection. See **Chapter 9.3 and 4.** →

Provide the best water quality you can and a varied diet. Prepare the specimens and examine for bacteria according to **Chart 21.**

NO ↓

B. The liver is greenish. → YES →

The bile duct is inflamed or obstructed. The bile is trapped in the liver and gives it the green color. →

This is probably an isolated case. The other fish do not need any treatment.

NO ↓

C. Small cysts (1 to 1.5mm) appear on and in the liver. → YES →

Probably metacercarial cysts. See **Chapter 7.3.** →

Prepare specimen and confirm the diagnosis by microscopic examination.

NO ↓

D. Small white nodules appear on the liver. → YES →

These can be sporozoan, tubercular or *Ichthyophonus* cysts. →

Prepare a mount of the cysts and examine at 50 X. See **Charts 20 and 21.**

NO ↓

E. Small eggs are seen in the squash mount of liver tissue (very rare). → YES →

Blood flukes may be affecting your fish. See **Chapter 7.3.** →

Prepare a mount. See part D in **Chart 7a.**

NO ↓

Go to **Chart 13.**

Carefully remove the gallbladder and position it on the slide before you puncture it.

**Chart 13
Gallbladder**

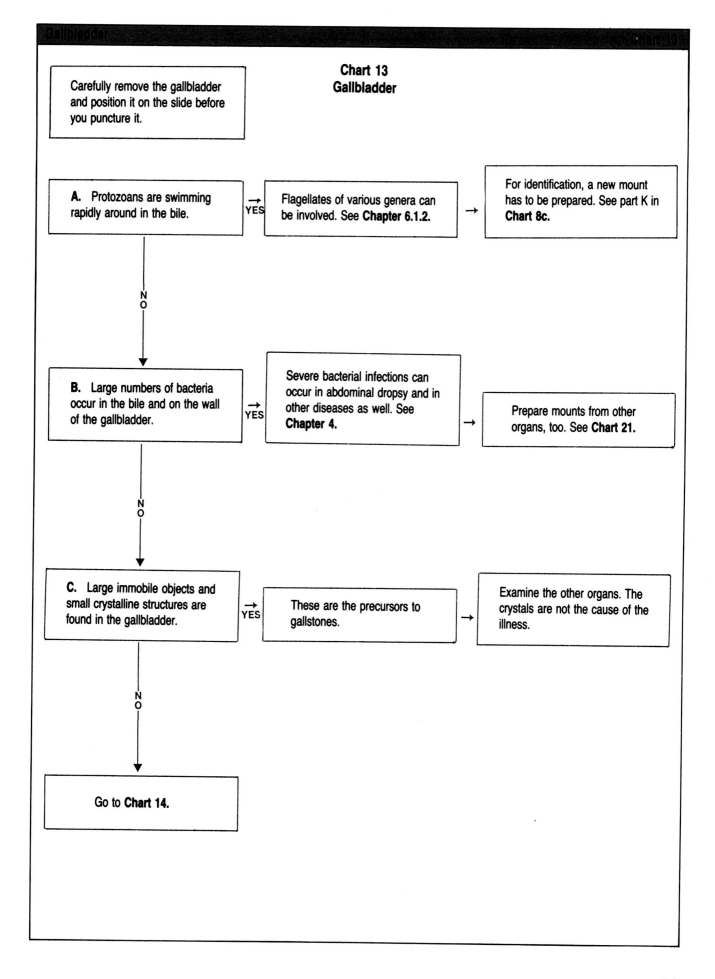

A. Protozoans are swimming rapidly around in the bile.

→ YES Flagellates of various genera can be involved. See **Chapter 6.1.2.**

→ For identification, a new mount has to be prepared. See part K in **Chart 8c.**

NO

B. Large numbers of bacteria occur in the bile and on the wall of the gallbladder.

→ YES Severe bacterial infections can occur in abdominal dropsy and in other diseases as well. See **Chapter 4.**

→ Prepare mounts from other organs, too. See **Chart 21.**

NO

C. Large immobile objects and small crystalline structures are found in the gallbladder.

→ YES These are the precursors to gallstones.

→ Examine the other organs. The crystals are not the cause of the illness.

NO

Go to **Chart 14.**

**Chart 14a
Intestines**

After you have prepared mounts of the intestines and their contents, interpret them according to this chart.

The fish is affected by acanthocephalans. See **Chapter 7.6.**

→ Do not feed with live water fleas. Deep-frozen ones are all right. Treat according to method **C24**. See part G in **Chart 8b**.

Photograph No. 26

A. The intestines contain opaque worms possessing a retractible proboscis or trunk completely covered with hooking structures. See Photograph No. 99.

YES

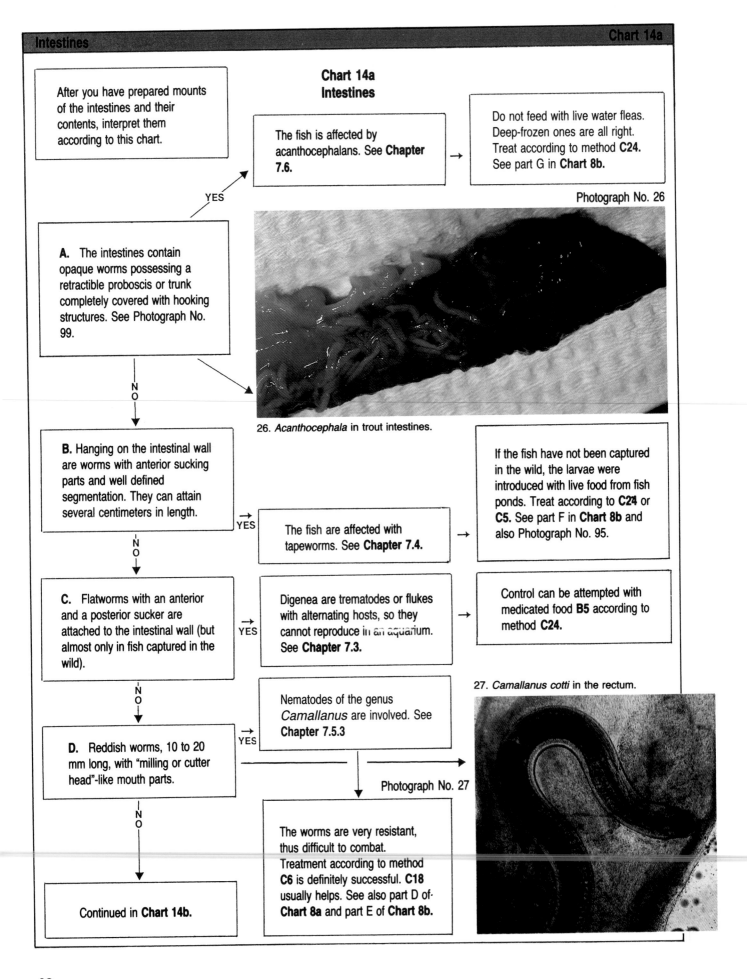

26. *Acanthocephala* in trout intestines.

NO

B. Hanging on the intestinal wall are worms with anterior sucking parts and well defined segmentation. They can attain several centimeters in length.

YES →

The fish are affected with tapeworms. See **Chapter 7.4.**

→ If the fish have not been captured in the wild, the larvae were introduced with live food from fish ponds. Treat according to **C24** or **C5**. See part F in **Chart 8b** and also Photograph No. 95.

NO

C. Flatworms with an anterior and a posterior sucker are attached to the intestinal wall (but almost only in fish captured in the wild).

YES →

Digenea are trematodes or flukes with alternating hosts, so they cannot reproduce in an aquarium. See **Chapter 7.3.**

→ Control can be attempted with medicated food **B5** according to method **C24**.

NO

27. *Camallanus cotti* in the rectum.

D. Reddish worms, 10 to 20 mm long, with "milling or cutter head"-like mouth parts.

YES →

Nematodes of the genus *Camallanus* are involved. See **Chapter 7.5.3**

Photograph No. 27

NO

Continued in **Chart 14b.**

The worms are very resistant, thus difficult to combat. Treatment according to method **C6** is definitely successful. **C18** usually helps. See also part D of **Chart 8a** and part E of **Chart 8b.**

Chart 14b
Intestines (continued)

Continued from Chart 14a

E. Long, very thin worms (up to 20mm long) move slowly in the intestines. Many eggs appear, too, with female specimens.

YES →

Capillarians are involved. See **Chapters 7.5** and **7.5.1.**

→

Examine the feces of the other fish to determine whether nematode eggs are present. Treat according to methods **C6** and **C5.** See also part H in **Chart 8b.**

NO

F. In cysts (250-350 u) embedded in the intestinal wall, curled-up worms move very slowly.

YES →

You have found encapsulated nematode larvae. See **Chapter 7.5** and Photograph No. 34 in **Chart 20.**

→

Treatment is not necessary.

NO

G. Large, thick worms (1 to 4mm) wriggle in the intestine. Only discus fish are known to have these.

YES →

These oxyurids have not been precisely identified. See **Chapter 7.5.2** and Photograph No. 98.

→

Look for eggs in the feces of the other fish. Treatment is by means of medicated food according to method **C6** or **C5.** See also part I in **Chart 8c.**

NO

H. Relatively large protozoans (100 u), which swim around in the intestinal contents, have slightly angled-off round anterior ends and a posterior end drawn out to a point.

YES →

The discus parasite *Protoopalina symphysodonis* has been found only in discus fish. See **Chapter 6.1.4.**

→

Treatment according to method **C19** quickly kills the flagellates. See also part L in **Chart 8d.**

NO

Continued in Chart 14c.

Chart 14C
Intestines (continued)

Continued from Chart 14b

I. Tiny protozoans (8 to 24u) move around very fast in the intestinal contents.

→ **YES** → The fish's intestines are infected with flagellates. See **Chapter 6.1.2.**

→ You can identify the flagellates with part K in **Chart 8c.**

↓ **NO**

K. Elongated cysts with clearly visible nucleus are seen in the intestinal wall.

→ **YES** → These are foreign bodies which have penetrated into the intestinal wall and been encapsulated there (e.g., *Cyclops* bristles). See **Chapter 9.1**

→ Do not feed *Cyclops* to fish which are not accustomed to them.

Photograph No. 28

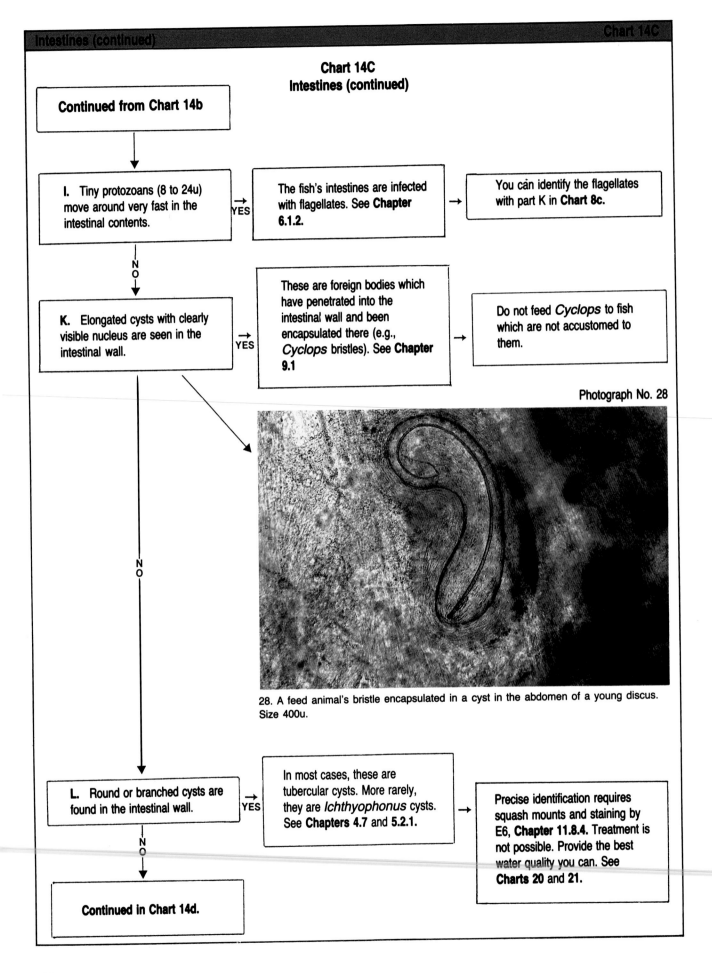

28. A feed animal's bristle encapsulated in a cyst in the abdomen of a young discus. Size 400u.

↓ **NO**

L. Round or branched cysts are found in the intestinal wall.

→ **YES** → In most cases, these are tubercular cysts. More rarely, they are *Ichthyophonus* cysts. See **Chapters 4.7** and **5.2.1.**

→ Precise identification requires squash mounts and staining by E6, **Chapter 11.8.4.** Treatment is not possible. Provide the best water quality you can. See **Charts 20** and **21.**

↓ **NO**

Continued in Chart 14d.

**Chart 14d
Intestines (concluded)**

Continued from Chart 14c

M. Reddish spots appear in the intestinal wall. At high magnification, blood cells can be recognized.

YES → This involves enteritis or viral infection. See **Chapters 93** and **4.5.**

→ Prepare a mount and examine it for bacteria. See **Chart 21.**

Photograph No. 29

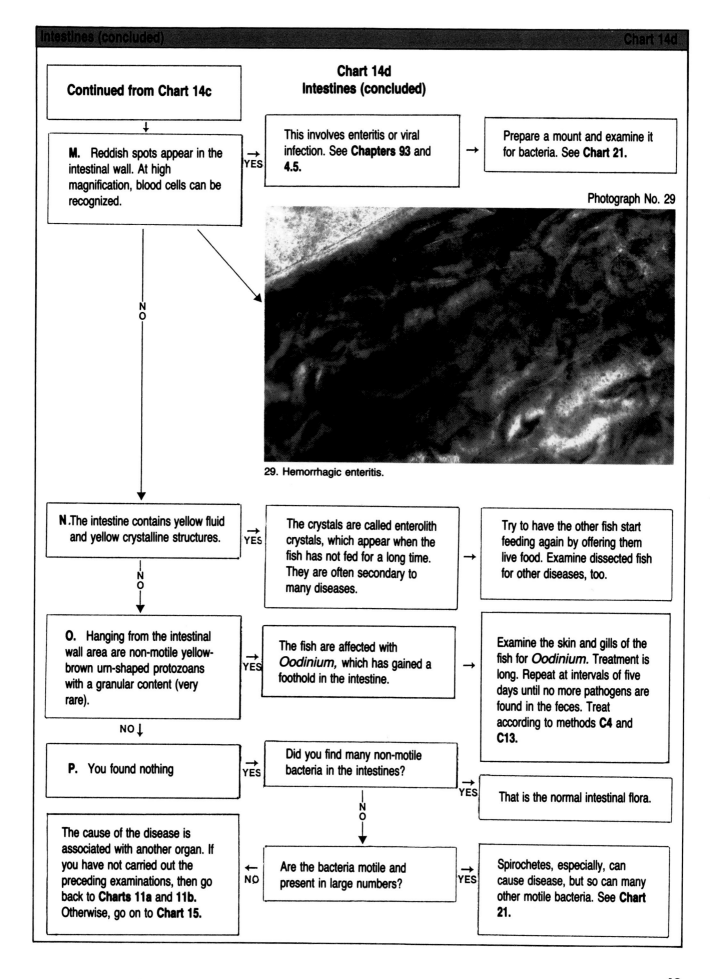

29. Hemorrhagic enteritis.

NO

N. The intestine contains yellow fluid and yellow crystalline structures.

YES → The crystals are called enterolith crystals, which appear when the fish has not fed for a long time. They are often secondary to many diseases.

→ Try to have the other fish start feeding again by offering them live food. Examine dissected fish for other diseases, too.

NO

O. Hanging from the intestinal wall area are non-motile yellow-brown urn-shaped protozoans with a granular content (very rare).

YES → The fish are affected with *Oodinium,* which has gained a foothold in the intestine.

→ Examine the skin and gills of the fish for *Oodinium.* Treatment is long. Repeat at intervals of five days until no more pathogens are found in the feces. Treat according to methods **C4** and **C13.**

NO

P. You found nothing

YES → Did you find many non-motile bacteria in the intestines?

YES → That is the normal intestinal flora.

NO

The cause of the disease is associated with another organ. If you have not carried out the preceding examinations, then go back to **Charts 11a** and **11b.** Otherwise, go on to **Chart 15.**

← NO Are the bacteria motile and present in large numbers?

YES → Spirochetes, especially, can cause disease, but so can many other motile bacteria. See **Chart 21.**

Chart 15
Spleen, Heart and Gonads

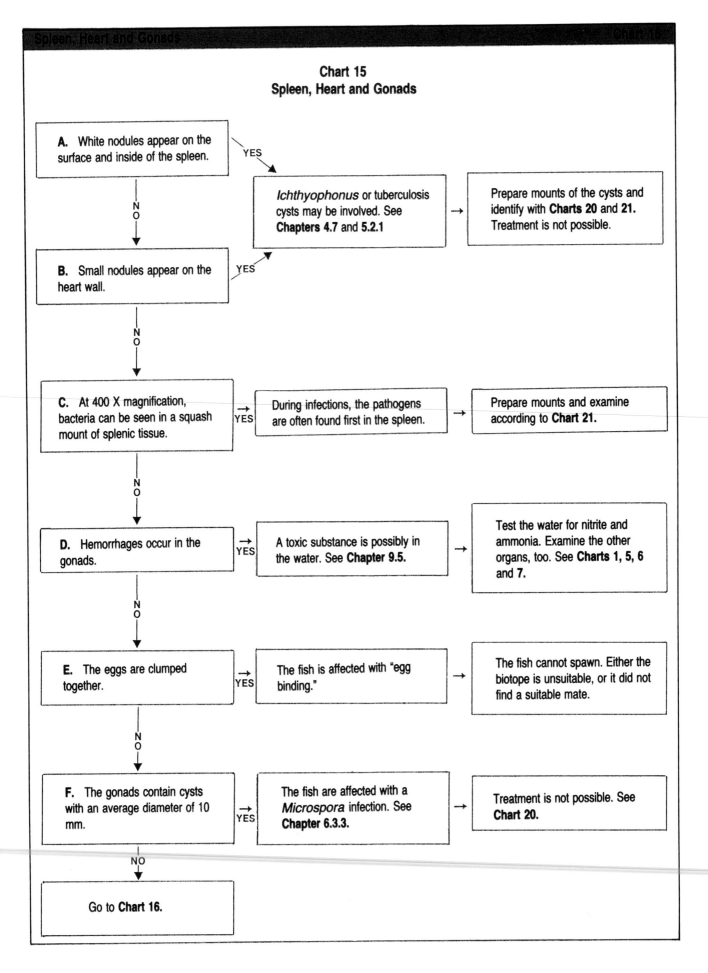

A. White nodules appear on the surface and inside of the spleen.

YES →

Ichthyophonus or tuberculosis cysts may be involved. See **Chapters 4.7** and **5.2.1**

→ Prepare mounts of the cysts and identify with **Charts 20** and **21**. Treatment is not possible.

NO ↓

B. Small nodules appear on the heart wall.

YES →

NO ↓

C. At 400 X magnification, bacteria can be seen in a squash mount of splenic tissue.

YES →

During infections, the pathogens are often found first in the spleen.

→ Prepare mounts and examine according to **Chart 21**.

NO ↓

D. Hemorrhages occur in the gonads.

YES →

A toxic substance is possibly in the water. See **Chapter 9.5**.

→ Test the water for nitrite and ammonia. Examine the other organs, too. See **Charts 1, 5, 6** and **7**.

NO ↓

E. The eggs are clumped together.

YES →

The fish is affected with "egg binding."

→ The fish cannot spawn. Either the biotope is unsuitable, or it did not find a suitable mate.

NO ↓

F. The gonads contain cysts with an average diameter of 10 mm.

YES →

The fish are affected with a *Microspora* infection. See **Chapter 6.3.3**.

→ Treatment is not possible. See **Chart 20**.

NO ↓

Go to **Chart 16**.

Chart 16
Air Bladder or Swim Bladder

A. The air bladder contains purulent fluid. Large numbers of bacteria are found in the fluid and the wall.

→ YES This involves a bacterial infection, usually as a result of an inflammation.

→ Examine the other organs, too. See **Chart 21.**

NO ↓

B. The wall of the air bladder is hardened.

→ YES The air bladder is inflamed.

→ Raise the water temperature by 3 to 5°C for five days.

NO ↓

C. Round cysts of various sizes (usually smaller than 1 mm) occur in the wall of the air bladder.

→ YES The fish are affected by the sporozoan *Eimeria.* See **Chapter 6.3.1.**

→ Examine the other organs, too, for cysts. Treatment, according to method **C22,** is only rarely successful. See **Chart 20.**

NO ↓

D. Large inclusions (up to 10mm) occur in the wall of the air bladder.

→ YES The fish is affected with *Microspora.* See **Chapter 6.3.3** .

→ Treatment is not possible. Examine the other organs, too. See **Chart 20.**

NO ↓

E. The anterior part of the air bladder, the part towards the abdomen, is inflamed. These fish were "standing on their heads," or else lying on the bottom.

→ YES A bacterial infection is the cause. See **Chapter 3.11** .

→ Treatment, by method **C26,** usually works, but is not successful in all cases.

NO ↓

Photograph No. 30

Go to **Chart 17.**

30. Inflammation of the air bladder in a *Symphysodon discus.*

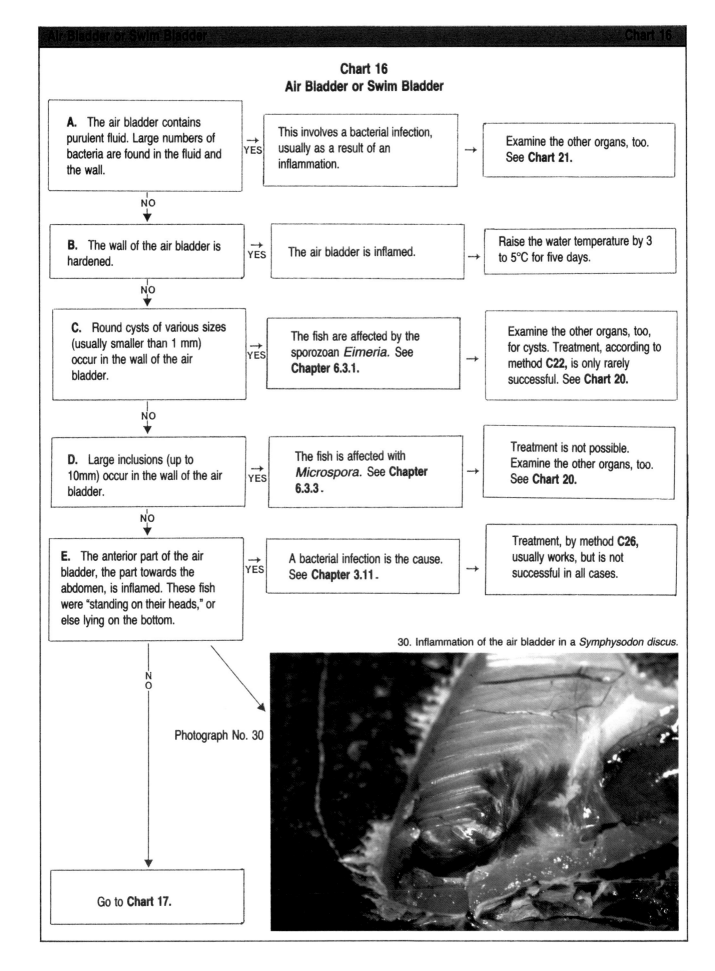

Chart 17
Kidneys

A. Small, motile protozoans are found in a squash mount of kidney tissue.

→ YES →

This involves flagellates which were transported by the blood to the kidneys.

→

Since you have already examined the intestine and gallbladder, you are now familiar with the flagellates. The other fish are most certainly infected as well, so rapid treatment is necessary. See **Chapter 6.1. Use methods C8 and C19.**

↓ NO

B. Large numbers of bacteria are found in the tissues. Also, hemorrhages often occur.

→ YES →

When bacteria gain entry to the kidneys, the rest of the body is certainly also affected.

→

Examine the spleen and liver, too. See **Charts 21** and **7**, as well as methods **C21, C25, C22, A5, A6** and **A1.**

↓ NO

C. Cysts of various sizes occur in the kidney tissue.

→ YES →

Tubercular and *Ichthyophonus* cysts are often found in the kidney.

→

Refer to **Charts 20** and **21** for definite identification. Treatment is not possible.

↓ NO

D. The kidney tubules contain crystals and inclusion bodies.

→ YES →

Organic substances often coat the crystals, so that multilayered structures are kidney stones. See Photograph No. 31 in this chart.

→

There are several causes of kidney stones in fish, i.e., medications and calcium crystallize or settle out in the kidneys.

↓ NO

Photograph No. 31

Go to **Chart 18.**

31. Sediment in the kidney tubules. (Phase contrast photograph.)

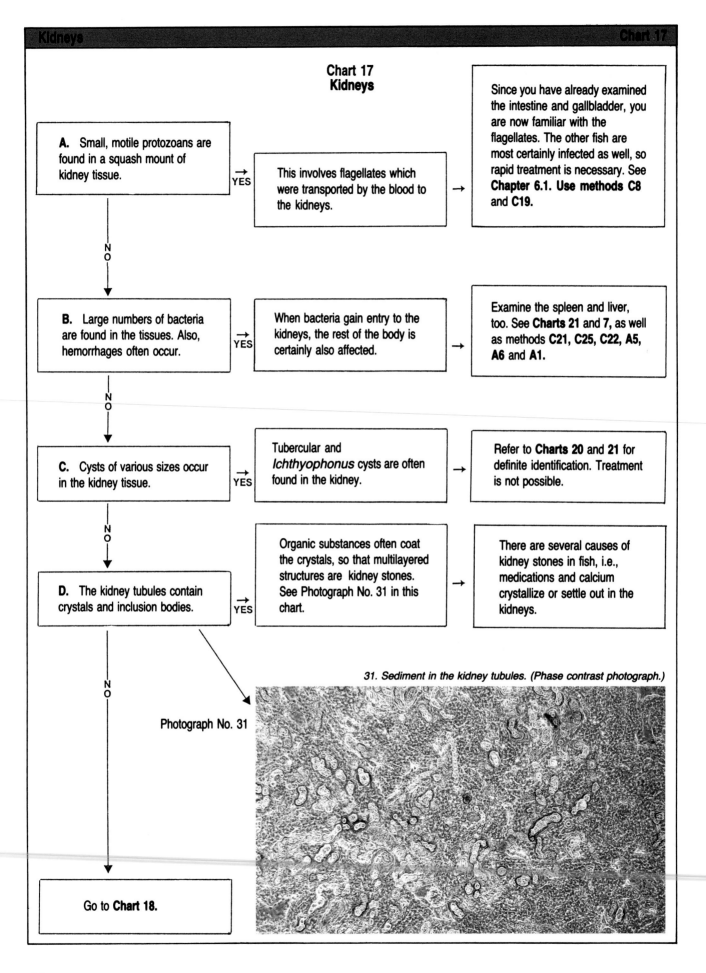

Chart 18
Brain and Muscle

A. Cysts of various sizes and dark contents are found in squash mounts of brain substance.

YES →

Probably tubercular cysts. See **Chapter 4.7.**

→

Prepare double squash mounts and examine according to **Chart 21.**

B. Often only thicker, contrasty areas are found in a squash mount of brain tissues.

YES →

NO ↓

C. Muscle mounts contain cysts with worms and larvae.

YES →

The fish is the intermediate host for these worms. See **Chapter 7.3.**

→

Fish captured in the wild are often infected with these. If larvae appear in offspring bred in the aquarium, then they were brought in with their intermediate hosts. Do not feed live foods obtained from fish ponds. See **Chart 20.**

NO ↓

D. The musculature is soft and white in places, and contains cysts which release many spores when pressed in a squash mount.

YES →

Sporozoan cysts of the genus *Pleistophora* are involved.

→

Treatment may be attempted with method **C22**, but is only rarely successful. For precise identification, see **Chart 20.**

NO ↓

Go to Chart 19.

Photograph No. 32

32. *Plistophora* cysts in a squashed muscle mount from a *Macropodus chinensis*.

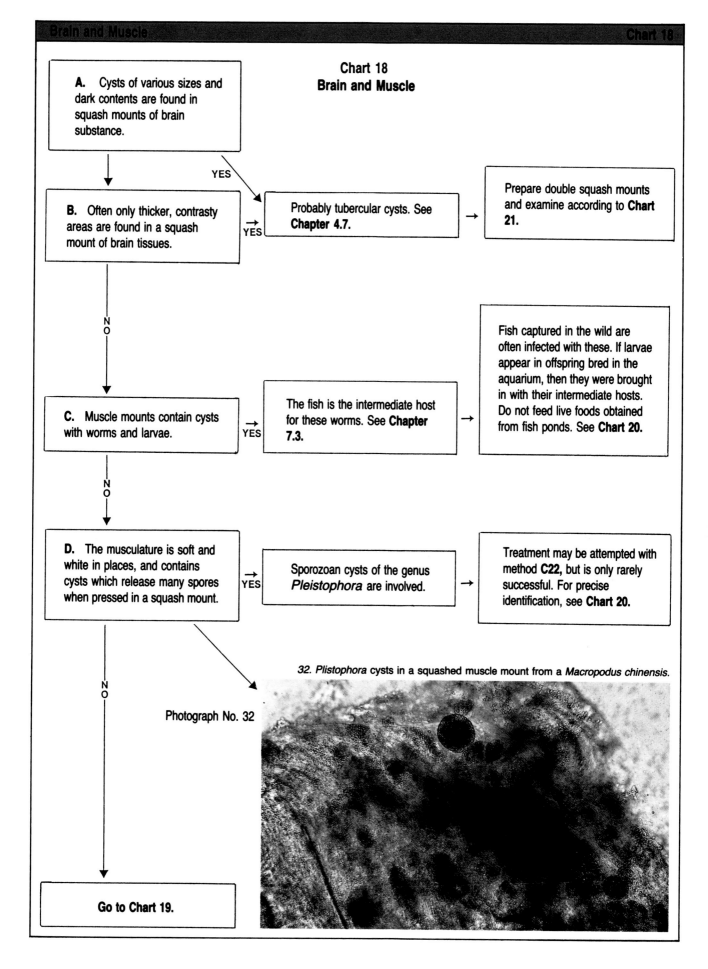

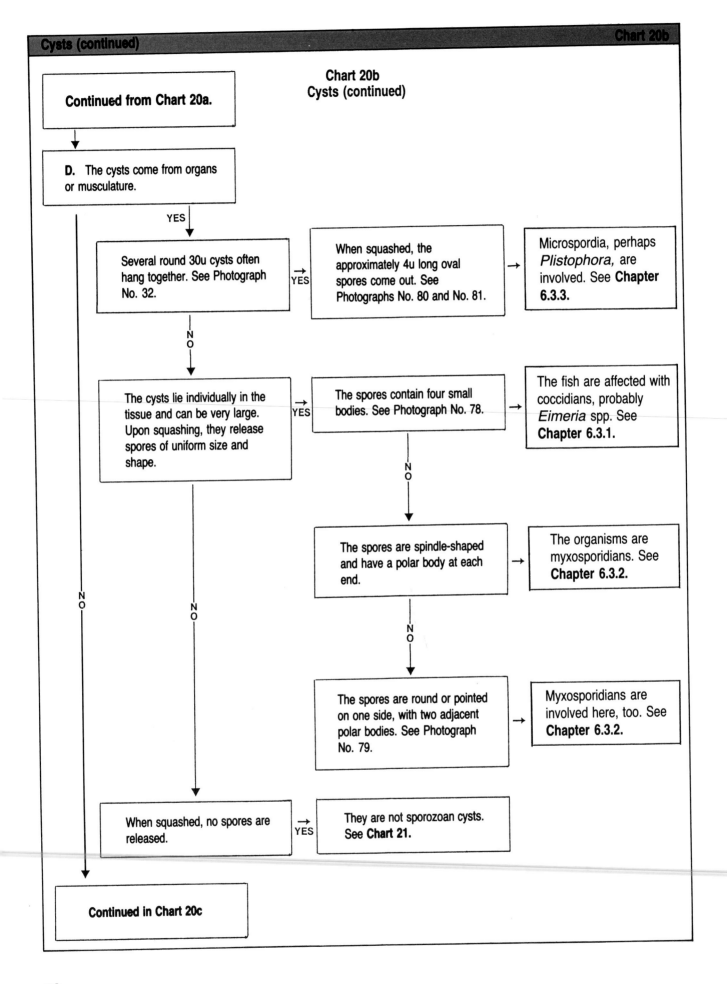

Chart 20b
Cysts (continued)

Continued from Chart 20a.

D. The cysts come from organs or musculature.

YES

Several round 30u cysts often hang together. See Photograph No. 32.

YES → When squashed, the approximately 4u long oval spores come out. See Photographs No. 80 and No. 81. → Microspordia, perhaps *Plistophora,* are involved. See **Chapter 6.3.3.**

NO

The cysts lie individually in the tissue and can be very large. Upon squashing, they release spores of uniform size and shape.

YES → The spores contain four small bodies. See Photograph No. 78. → The fish are affected with coccidians, probably *Eimeria* spp. See **Chapter 6.3.1.**

NO

The spores are spindle-shaped and have a polar body at each end. → The organisms are myxosporidians. See **Chapter 6.3.2.**

NO

The spores are round or pointed on one side, with two adjacent polar bodies. See Photograph No. 79. → Myxosporidians are involved here, too. See **Chapter 6.3.2.**

When squashed, no spores are released. YES → They are not sporozoan cysts. See **Chart 21.**

NO

Continued in Chart 20c

Chart 20c
Cysts (continued)

Continued from Chart 20b.

E. The cysts come from a lesion or a thickened area of tissue. → YES → The cysts are encapsulated in light-colored tissues. No structures are visible inside. They range in color from light to dark brown. See Photograph No. 61 → YES → Tuberculosis is probably involved here. See **Chart 21.**

NO ↓

The tissue is firm, and squashing expresses only a few cells. Extensively covered with black pigment cells. → YES → Probably a malignant tumor, a melanosarcoma, which is common in livebearing cyprinodonts but rare in other fish. See also Photograph No. 106 → Observe the other fish closely. See **Chapter 9.1, Charts 3** and **4b (part D).**

NO ↓

The inside tissue is decomposed and viscous. The lesion can be open or closed. → YES → The lesion is purulent. Prepare a mount and examine it for bacteria. See **Chart 21.**

F. Over the course of several weeks, a domed swelling has formed under the skin. → YES → After the skin is cut open, a firm, spheroid structure can be removed which does not adhere to the musculature. → YES → Such benign tumors can also form on organs. They are not dangerous to the other fish. See **Chapter 9.1.**

NO ↓

Photograph No. 35.

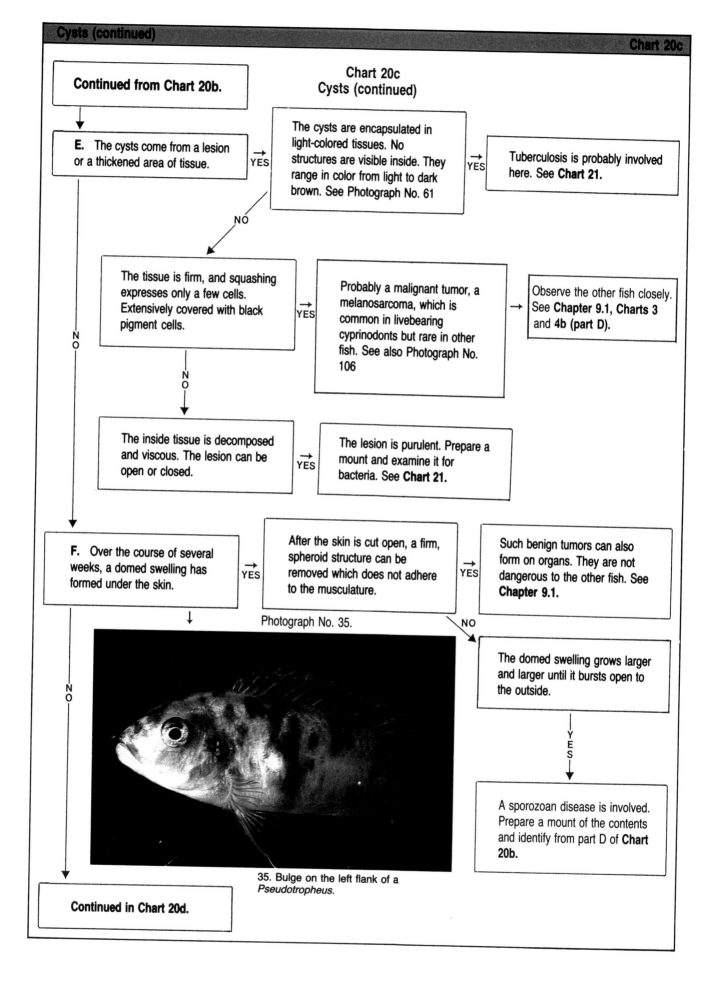

35. Bulge on the left flank of a *Pseudotropheus.*

NO → The domed swelling grows larger and larger until it bursts open to the outside.

YES ↓

A sporozoan disease is involved. Prepare a mount of the contents and identify from part D of **Chart 20b.**

Continued in Chart 20d.

51

Chart 20d
Cysts (concluded)

Continued from Chart 20c.

G. Isolated or many irregularly elongated cysts are found in the intestinal wall. A clearly visible foreign body is visible inside.

→ YES: Sharp fragments of food have penetrated into the intestinal wall, where they have been encapsulated by the surrounding tissue. *Cyclops* bristles are usually involved, rarely mosquito larvae. See Photograph No. 28. → Do not feed your fish that food any more.

↓ NO

H. Cysts measuring 50 to 500u are found in the organs. Dark, nonmotile contents. The cysts are surrounded by light tissue. See Photograph No. 61.

→ YES: Tuberculosis or *Ichthyophonus* is involved. → Prepare double squash mounts and examine for bacteria. See **Chart 21.**

↓ NO

I. The cysts are irregular and branched, or very small.

→ YES: Tiny foreign bodies may have been encapsulated, or tubercular cysts may be involved. → Prepare double squash mounts and examine for bacteria. See **Chart 21.**

↓ NO

K. Small, round cysts (measuring 0.8mm at most) are found on the gill filaments.

→ YES: Squashing does not express any spores, just small (0.3 to 1u) coccus-shaped pathogens. → Chlamydia are the cause. These tiny spheroid bacteria can be seen only in well-prepared mounts under a good microscope. See **Chart 21.**

↓ NO

Go on to Chart 21.

Chart 21a
Bacteria

You have found bacteria in a smear or squash mount. Now, with water, prepare an extremely dilute mount and examine at 400 to 800 X magnification. Dark field or phase contrast is very helpful. In contrast to other organisms, bacteria are not identified merely by size and appearance. Costly methods are necessary to identify them. Cultures must be seeded and the growth of colonies observed on various kinds of culture media. Then the cultured bacteria can be classified according to their metabolic characteristics. The culture of bacteria is not harmless, so for this reason it should be carried out only by trained specialists in specially equipped laboratories. In that respect, then, this chart is not an actual diagnostic chart, but rather an aid in deciding on the best selection of medication. (That is, precise diagnosis is not always necessary before treatment can be started.)

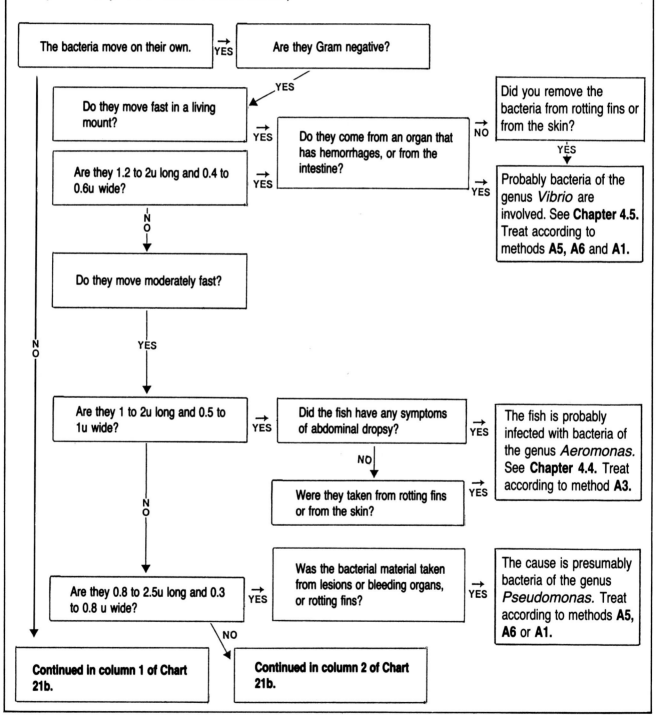

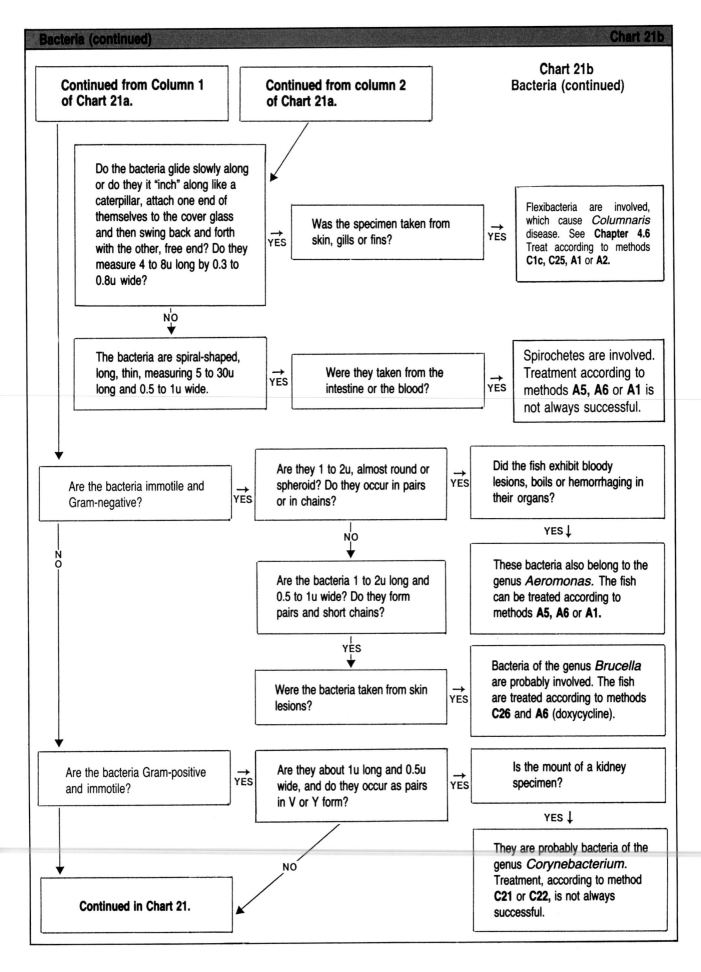

Chart 21b
Bacteria (continued)

Continued from Column 1 of Chart 21a.

Continued from column 2 of Chart 21a.

Do the bacteria glide slowly along or do they it "inch" along like a caterpillar, attach one end of themselves to the cover glass and then swing back and forth with the other, free end? Do they measure 4 to 8u long by 0.3 to 0.8u wide?

→ YES → Was the specimen taken from skin, gills or fins? → YES → Flexibacteria are involved, which cause *Columnaris* disease. See **Chapter 4.6** Treat according to methods **C1c**, **C25**, **A1** or **A2**.

NO ↓

The bacteria are spiral-shaped, long, thin, measuring 5 to 30u long and 0.5 to 1u wide. → YES → Were they taken from the intestine or the blood? → YES → Spirochetes are involved. Treatment according to methods **A5**, **A6** or **A1** is not always successful.

Are the bacteria immotile and Gram-negative? → YES → Are they 1 to 2u, almost round or spheroid? Do they occur in pairs or in chains? → YES → Did the fish exhibit bloody lesions, boils or hemorrhaging in their organs?

YES ↓

NO ↓

Are the bacteria 1 to 2u long and 0.5 to 1u wide? Do they form pairs and short chains?

These bacteria also belong to the genus *Aeromonas*. The fish can be treated according to methods **A5**, **A6** or **A1**.

YES ↓

Were the bacteria taken from skin lesions? → YES → Bacteria of the genus *Brucella* are probably involved. The fish are treated according to methods **C26** and **A6** (doxycycline).

NO ↓

Are the bacteria Gram-positive and immotile? → YES → Are they about 1u long and 0.5u wide, and do they occur as pairs in V or Y form? → YES → Is the mount of a kidney specimen?

YES ↓

NO →

They are probably bacteria of the genus *Corynebacterium*. Treatment, according to method **C21** or **C22**, is not always successful.

Continued in Chart 21.

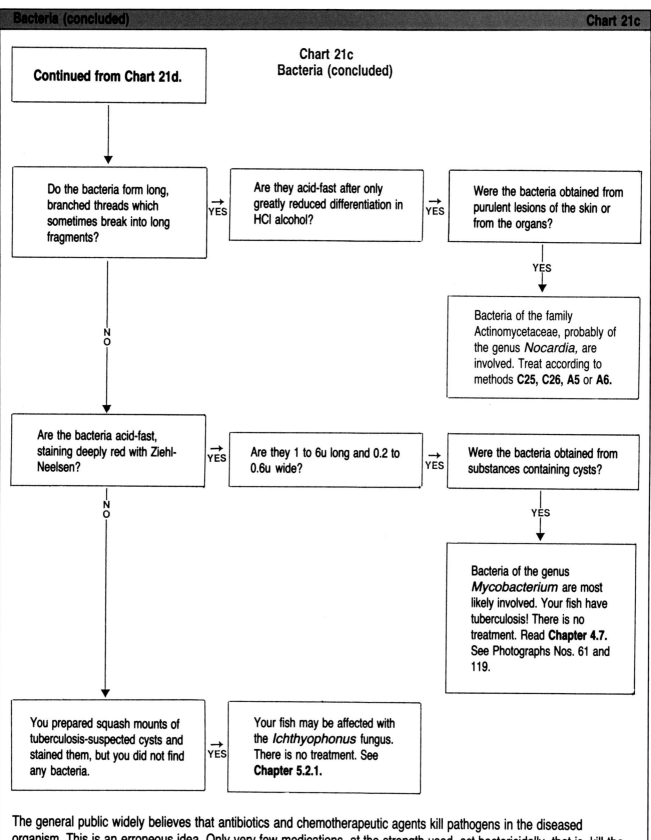

Chart 21c
Bacteria (concluded)

Continued from Chart 21d.

Do the bacteria form long, branched threads which sometimes break into long fragments?

→ YES → Are they acid-fast after only greatly reduced differentiation in HCl alcohol?

→ YES → Were the bacteria obtained from purulent lesions of the skin or from the organs?

↓ YES

Bacteria of the family Actinomycetaceae, probably of the genus *Nocardia,* are involved. Treat according to methods **C25, C26, A5** or **A6.**

NO

Are the bacteria acid-fast, staining deeply red with Ziehl-Neelsen?

→ YES → Are they 1 to 6u long and 0.2 to 0.6u wide?

→ YES → Were the bacteria obtained from substances containing cysts?

↓ YES

Bacteria of the genus *Mycobacterium* are most likely involved. Your fish have tuberculosis! There is no treatment. Read **Chapter 4.7.** See Photographs Nos. 61 and 119.

NO

You prepared squash mounts of tuberculosis-suspected cysts and stained them, but you did not find any bacteria.

→ YES → Your fish may be affected with the *Ichthyophonus* fungus. There is no treatment. See **Chapter 5.2.1.**

The general public widely believes that antibiotics and chemotherapeutic agents kill pathogens in the diseased organism. This is an erroneous idea. Only very few medications, at the strength used, act bactericidally, that is, kill the bacteria. Most act bacteriostatically, that is, merely inhibit the growth of the bacteria. That means, in practical terms, that the bacteria attacking the organism will be impeded in their multiplication, thereby allowing the body's own resistance to recuperate and then destroy the bacteria. A fish whose resistance is completely exhausted will not be returned to health even with antibiotics, but will continue to sicken and finally die.

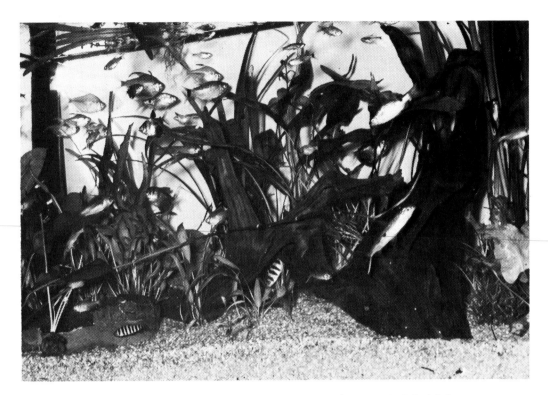

The basic task of good aquarium management is to see to it that fishes are not subjected to stressful conditions. Under conditions of prolonged stress, even the healthiest of fishes will eventually succumb. Fortunately, the most important causes of stress in the aquarium are entirely controllable by the aquarist, who can rely on a combination of good equipment and good aquarium management practices to reduce stress.

Chapter 2
RECOGNIZING DISEASES

2.1. Fish Under Stress

Not only human beings, but also fish suffer from stress. Aquarium fish, especially, can be exposed to many kinds of stress. The cause usually is environmental.

Stress factors for fish in an aquarium are: frequent fluctuations in water temperature; water chemistry alien to the species placed in it; chemical substances (fertilizer, medication); polluted water; crowding; water saturated with excrement; improper diet; transfers; moving, overly strong water circulation; and quarantine in unsuitable tanks. A fish's fear also is a stress factor that should not be underestimated. Frequent handling, netting, or even your own rapid movement by the tank can trigger anxiety. Intraspecific fighting for a place in the pecking order means intense stress for the inferior fish if the tank is too small and hiding refuges too few. Extreme stress can lead to shock and death of the fish.

Fish are often exposed to stress from substances in the water. For a certain period of time a fish can maintain its homeostasis (body equilibrium) by adapting to the changing factors. When this is no longer possible, a state of exhaustion sets in, ending in death. Wedemeyer (1970, 1974) was able to demonstrate that stress directly weakens resistance to infections. The result is often an outbreak of disease caused by latent stages of parasites or by organisms in the aquarium (Chapter 6).

Overpopulation severely stresses the inhabitants of the aquarium. Even with good filtration, the water is increasingly polluted with the accumulation of wastes. The fish get in each other's way and lack sufficient hiding places. A guideline for the optimal population of a tank is often quoted as five liters of water per fish (1 liter = 1.06 quart). Therefore, a 100-liter aquarium can house 20 fish. Large or small fish? This kind of calculation leaves something to be desired.

Good results have been obtained with the following figures, with which population limits are set according to the quantity of water per fish length:

Fish Size	Amount of Water per 1 cm of Fish Length
under 2 cm	1 liter
2 to 5 cm	1.5 liters
6 to 9 cm	2 liters
10 to 13 cm	3 liters
14 cm and over	4 liters

When setting up a tank with young fish, the calculation should be based upon the anticipated adult length, of course. With these guidelines, a good filtering system, and regular changes of water, metabolic wastes will not seriously burden the water, unless you systematically overfeed. Beware of those aquarium fish foods that claim "doesn't cloud the water." All foods cloud the water if uneaten . . . and most foods cloud the water after they've been eaten if the fish don't digest them. If your tank gets cloudy, change the fish food and feed less.

2.2. Prevention of Diseases

To keep fish in an aquarium healthy and to provide for their long life, the guidelines in this chapter must be taken to heart so as to prevent disease and, by the appropriate means, avoid introduction of diseases. Therefore, new arrivals should be quarantined before introduction into the aquarium (Chapter 2.4). Use several catch-nets, ideally a separate one for each tank. A bucketful of concentrated disinfectant solution serves for the sterilization of used nets and other items that come into contact with aquarium water (Chapter 10, substances D_1 to D_6). These items should be kept from the bucketful of disinfectant except when being used, but they must be rinsed off in clean water before use. Neither these items nor your hands should be taken out of one tank and dipped into another tank without first disinfecting them and then rinsing them. This cuts down on the transmission of disease organisms from one tank to another. Nor should water itself be transferred from one tank to another. Besides regular daily observation when raising young fish, sanitary check-ups should be carried out at least every two weeks. This includes primarily microscopic examination (at 50 to 200X) of fresh feces.

Plants that were not grown or kept in fish-free tanks can bring parasites into the aquarium. As a rule, plants from nurseries can be considered free of disease-causing organisms. Plants that were in contact with fish can be disinfected in an alum solution (Chapter 10, method D_4).

In summary, it should be noted that the successful prevention of disease depends to a large extent upon how religiously the maintenance is carried out and the precautionary measures adhered to.

Regular water changes are obligatory. It is better to do it often with a little water than infrequently with a lot of water. Support the biological self-cleansing processes in the water by providing active biological filtration. The fish that lives under healthy conditions is in a better position to resist even the more aggressive parasites. Since the aquarium represents a limited cosmos, adult parasites as well as their larvae and free-swimming forms have a much better chance of finding a fish than they would in the wild.

2.3. Poisoning and Disease

Recognition of the cause of a fish disease is the prerequisite for successful treatment. Basically, we have to differentiate between diseases caused by pathogens and diseases whose causes reside in the fish itself or in its environment. The latter—fish and environment—include hereditary diseases, deformities, toxicity, injuries, and improper diet. The

recognition and control, as far as is possible, of these causes are described in Chapter 9. Diseases caused by pathogens, however, are more frequent. Pathogens are all living organisms that can cause disease.

If the fish act abnormally, the first step is to find out if all fish or only one species of fish or only a few fish act this way. If the symptoms appear within a brief period in all the fish, or if at least the more sensitive species exhibit the same abnormal behavior, poisoning is highly probable. This can be expressed in the most varied ways. During and after the poisoning, you may observe disrupted equilibrium, paralysis, twitching, cramps, darting about the tank at the slightest stimulus and then bumping into things because of a decreased sense of perception, rapid breathing, gasping for air just under the surface of the water, fading of coloration, discoloration of the gills and fins, red spots on the body, whitish cloudiness of the skin, or increased secretion of mucus.

Depending upon the kind of toxin involved, removal of the cause may bring improvement. If a powerful toxin has affected the fish, they can still succumb later, even in toxin-free water, from the delayed effects of the toxin.

Recognition of poisoning is very difficult when only slight traces of the toxin remain in the water. Damage then occurs only over the course of time. It has been observed, for example, that fish died of organ damage only at a mature age, while young fish were not affected. At times poisoning is expressed only by the sharp increase in the number of various ectoparasites.

Diseases caused primarily by pathogens rarely spread quickly to the whole population in well maintained aquariums. It is always just a few fish that are affected first, unless the whole tank has been newly filled with fish that are already diseased. The observant aquarium hobbyist soon recognizes the change in behavior of a few fish, so there is still enough time to take countermeasures.

In order to recognize any change in the fish's behavior as pathological, the aquarium keeper must be very familiar with the lifestyle of his charges in a healthy state. This familiarity, of course, comes only with frequent observation. Behavioral changes that reveal diseases are not expressed in the same way in all species. Likewise, we cannot conclude from a change in behavior that the fish has a specific disease, for a certain change in behavior may have one or more of many different causes. Thus, staggering along, paler or darkened coloration, and clamped together fins are symptoms of exhaustion and extreme malaise possibly associated with internal damage. Likewise, extremely high or low pH values, heat, cold, and lack of oxygen could be the causes. Swimming on the side, disequilibrium, "standing on the head," and turning over suggest severe damage caused by an infection of the brain, air bladder, or labyrinth (organ of balance), or they can indicate the terminal stage of a disease.

Refusal of food, associated with standing apart from the other fish, timidity, darkening, and holes in the fins suggest intestinal endoparasites. If a fish does not react and is extremely lethargic, it may be affected with blood flagellates.

Bacterial infections of various internal organs lead to lethargy, fading of colors, staying apart from the others, darkening, refusal to feed, inflamed anus, slimy feces, often breathing rapidly, and pale gills.

If the fish rub against decorations and plants and twitch their fins vigorously or fold them together, then ectoparasites are affecting them. Spreading of the opercula, associated with rubbing and frequent, rapid protrusion of the mouth, indicates gill worms. Rapid breathing, however, is not a definite symptom of gill worms. The cause can also be a toxin in the water, lack of oxygen, improper pH, or another stressful factor. (See diagnostic charts in Chapter 1.)

2.4. Quarantine and Disinfection

A quarantine tank should be part of every serious aquarium keeper's equipment. It does not have to be very large, as long as it is adequate for the size and number of the fish to be observed in it (see under 2.2). The interior ar-rangement and water quality should match, if possible, that of the future home of the fish in the permanent aquarium. Make sure, however, that all of the decorative items can be removed for a short time when fish must be treated or caught.

As a rule, all new additions should be kept in quarantine for three to six weeks and their well-being checked daily. Three weeks is the minimum time to quarantin e fish that were raised in aquaria, for the development of many parasites can take two weeks before reaching a stage at which the signs of a disease become apparent. Five to six weeks are appropriate for fish captured in the wild and fish raised in ponds, which often harbor unrecognized parasites. During this time, transfer some water from the aquarium into the quarantine tank to start adapting the new fish to the microflora and microfauna of their future home. The second function of the quarantine tank is that of a hospital tank for fish suspected of being diseased. They can be observed for quite some time there without jeopardizing the other fish in the aquarium.

Diseases that are recognized late are difficult to treat. If the whole fish population should perish due to an epidemic, it is advisable to thoroughly disinfect both the aquarium and the quarantine tank. Destroy the plants. With pathogens higher on the evolutionary scale than bacteria and viruses, disinfection of plants with alum (Chapter 10, method D_4) can be considered. Decorative items, roots, rocks, gravel, and filter contents should be boiled one hour, without counting the warm-up time. Sterilize the empty aquarium and the non-boilable objects with a strong potassium permanganate solution as per D_1, K_{10}. Let the filter run without substrate so the container, pump, and tubing are disinfected at the same time. Set up the aquarium again after all the parts, including the tank, are thoroughly rinsed. Fill the filter with new substrate or the old, boiled substrate. After starting up, the filter again needs a running-in time of six weeks until adequate numbers of bacteria have built up.

2.5. Examination of Living Fish

When a fish falls sick and poisoning of the water can be eliminated as a possible cause, immediately transfer the fish to the quarantine tank. Examination begins with observation (Charts 1 to 4); a definite time every day must be devoted to it. Any irregularities observed must be recorded so that later on the whole course of the disease can be documented. Protocols such as the one presented below simplify the work and save time. You can prepare a master typewritten original and then make photocopies. These protocols can be kept for future reference. The form should also contain the "patient's" history, behavior, date of last water change, chemical quality of the water, last feeding, etc. The following key words can be modified according to individual needs. (The layman should not, under any circumstances, examine venomous fish!)

Behavioral changes usually appear in an advanced stage of disease, so that immediate treatment of the fish is called for. For that, trap the fish in a net against the wall of the aquarium and examine its skin closely with a magnifying glass (Charts 5 and 6). The larger parasites, like the carp louse and *Ichthyophthirius,* are easily recognized. Further examination requires that the fish be lifted briefly out of the water. The ocular reflex can now be tested. As shown in Photograph No. 36, the fish attempts, when rotated around the long axis, to keep looking horizontally, so rolls its eyes to

36. Healthy fish keep their eyes horizontal when the body is rotated around the long axis.

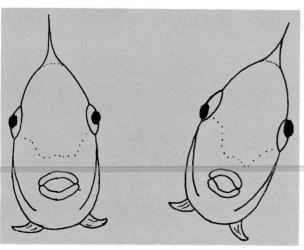

EXAMINATION

1. **Protocol number:** _____
2. **Date:** _____
3. **Species:** _____
4. **Sex:** _____
5. **Origin/Owner:** _____
6. **How Long Kept:** _____
7. **Water volume:** _____
8. **Population density:** _____
9. **Filtration:** _____
10. **Water values:** _____
11. **Feed/Diet:** _____
12. **Number dead:** _____
13. **At what intervals did they die?** ___
14. **In what species were the deaths?**
_____
15. **Behavior of sick fish:** _____
16. **Preventive measures:** _____
17. **Any treatment attempted:** _____
18. **Examination of the live fish**
    A. EXTERNAL DESCRIPTION: _____
    B. COLOR: _____
    C. SKIN SMEAR: _____
    D. FIN SMEAR: _____
    E. GILL SMEAR: _____
    F. FECES: _____
19. **Autopsy**
    A. SKIN SMEAR: _____
    B. FIN FRAGMENTS: _____
    C. SCALES: _____
    D. BLOOD: _____
    E. GILLS: _____
    F. BODY CAVITY: _____
    G. LIVER: _____
    H. GALLBLADDER: _____
    I. STOMACH: _____
    J. INTESTINES: _____
    K. SPLEEN: _____
    L. HEART: _____
    M. GONADS: _____
    N. AIR BLADDER: _____
    O. KIDNEYS: _____
    P. BRAIN: _____
    Q. MUSCULATURE: _____
20. **Diagnosis:** _____
21. **Therapy:** _____
22. **Therapeutic success:** _____

counteract being held on its side. If its eyes remain in a normal relationship to its body, then it is affected with a labyrinth problem.

In large fish, the tail reflex can be tested. For that test, hold the front part of the fish out of the water but in the normal swimming position. A fish that is still vigorous can hold its tail horizontal, but a weaker one lets the tail droop.

With a dissecting microscope, the skin can be carefully examined at 10X, 20X, and 30X, but take care that the fish are not kept out of water too long—three minutes maximum, if possible. To keep the fish from flopping off the table during any other examinations, wrap the fish in wet cotton cloth, but even then the time out of water should not exceed three minutes. Various parts of the body can be uncovered for examination and the taking of biopsy material. For that, run a scraper or knife lightly from the anterior to the posterior end of the area being tested to accumulate some slime. Take smears from the caudal peduncle, the angles formed at the bases of the pectoral fins, and the opercula (Photograph No. 37). Mix the

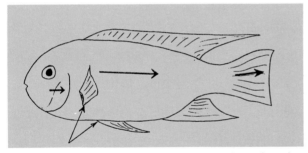

37. Smears are taken from flanks, opercula and angles between pectorals and body.

slime obtained from every smear separately with a drop of water on a separate microscope slide and cover with a cover slip (Chapter 11.4). Wipe the scraper (spatula) clean each time you scrape it over the fish. Now examine the mounts at 25X to 50X magnification. Large parasites will be easy to see. If higher magnification is necessary, press the cover slip lightly with the point of a dissecting needle and blot up (with blotter or filter paper) the water that is squeezed out at the sides of the cover slip. This is necessary because at high magnification a thick mount would require refocusing at many levels to get from the top to the bottom

of the specimen on the slide (Chapter 11.4), and even then, if the microscopic specimen becomes too thick it becomes too dense to see.

Further examination is best carried out on anesthetized fish (see Chapter 10, C_{20} for use of anesthesia), especially when lifting the operculum to take a gill smear; otherwise the fish wriggles so much that you can easily injure the gills. A fish can die from gill hemorrhages. Besides, the fish should be spared any unnecessary torment. As a rule, gill smears should be taken during every examination because many parasites can be found in this protected area.

Once the fish is wrapped in a wet cotton cloth, the gill area can be uncovered. Hold the fish's head firmly with the palm of the left hand, with the thumb and little finger hold the posterior area, and with the right palm hold the tail. With the fingernail of the ring finger or forefinger of the left hand, lift the operculum while leaving the thumb and forefinger of the right hand free to hold a small magnifying glass, forceps, or a pipette. Such a procedure, of course, is only possible with fish that are at least 10 cm (4 in) long. Use a magnifying glass to check the gill filaments for color and large parasites (Chart 7).

Any parasites found can be picked off with finely pointed forceps and prepared for microscopic examination (Chapter 11.6). Then obtain a smear from the gills. Be very careful because they can be more easily damaged than skin.

Another way of obtaining gill parasites is to hold a glass pipette (with its sharp tip melted a bit to make it blunt) on the gill arches and aspirate; all insecurely anchored parasites will be loosened and sucked up into the pipette, from which they can be transferred to a microscope slide and then looked for at 100X.

Even if the preceding methods were successful, the feces should also be examined (Chart 8). A fecal fragment may be obtained by repeatedly applying short, light squeezes to the abdomen. Transfer the feces to a microscope slide, swirl in a drop of water, and examine at 100X. *Protoopalina* and worms can now be seen. To see small objects such as worm eggs and flagellates, switch to 200-400X magnification. Keep the cover slip very close to the slide (by removing water with a blotter) to prevent overlayering of microscopic objects, which makes the slide too opaque to see through (Chapter 11.4).

Parasites that are not discovered by the methods described above are not numerous enough to present any danger to the fish. That could quickly change, however, if environmental and stress factors change. It is advisable to examine the feces of aquarium fish periodically, even if there is no disease suspected. Wait until a fish defecates, then pipette the feces up with a long pipette before it reaches the bottom of the tank. If the fecal thread hangs from the anus longer than ten minutes, it is limited in usefulness as a specimen, for many living parasites have already abandoned it. In addition, scavenger organisms (which the layman may think are parasites) soon begin to decompose the feces (Chapters 6.4.6 and 11.4, as well as Photographs Nos. 87, 88, 89, and 111 to 115). Many fish cannot defecate completely and for hours drag around a fecal thread—often whitish and slimy—that grows longer and longer. This indicates a serious intestinal disease, often a flagellate infection or enteritis (Chapter 6 and 9).

2.6. Humane Sacrificing of Fish

Occasionally fish become so seriously ill that recuperation seems impossible. In such a case it is more humane to quickly and painlessly sacrifice (a euphemism for "kill") the fish than to let it slowly die. It is unworthy of an animal lover to flush living fish down the toilet or to douse them with boiling water, both methods condemning the fish to a horrible death.

A brief consideration of animal protection laws on the Continent is appropriate here. Most laws require that animals be maintained (that is, those that are allowed to be maintained in captivity) as befits their species, with appropriate care and diet. No suffering, injuries, or pain may be inflicted upon the captive animal. Injury means physical and non-physical abuse, including starvation and overfeeding. Suffering means all lessening of well-being, such as overexcitement, overly restricted movement, hunger, temperatures that are too

high or low, overburdening of certain organs (such as goose liver paté), and keeping incompatible animals together.

The killing of vertebrates is prohibited, except for food and to put incurably damaged animals out of their misery. You must possess the required knowledge and skill before being allowed to kill an animal. The killing must be painfree and, when applicable, should be performed with the animal under anesthesia.

As a rule, young animals may not be killed. An exception is allowed when breeding fish—deformed fry or those exhibiting degenerative signs must be eliminated. These defective fry can be caught, sacrificed, and dissected for examination, thus lending some measure of control over the health of the fish and protecting the aquarium hobbyist from bad surprises such as sudden epidemics. Fish being raised in captivity and living in large schools are especially prone to massive parasitic attacks.

A head or neck incision is the most rapid way to dispatch a fish. Use scissors or a pointed scalpel to cut quickly and deeply behind the eyes and down to the upper edge of the operculum. This immediately destroys the brain. If the brain is needed for study, cut somewhat further behind and sever the vertebral column. After cutting into the neck, wait a few minutes until the brain has died and the head does not perceive any more stimuli. If you are not yet skilled or do not trust yourself in cutting quickly and deeply enough, then the fish can be heavily anesthetized beforehand. Once breathing is no longer apparent and the fish floats belly up, the anesthesia is deep enough so it will not feel the incision. As a rule, the humane procedure is to administer an overdose of anesthesia (Chapter 10, C_{20}) and then make certain with a neck incision.

Dissection is appropriate when a fish is visibly diseased but nothing is revealed from smears and fecal examination and no cure can be expected. Fish that die on their own are suitable for dissection only if they have not remained in the aquarium for more than 20 minutes, otherwise many parasites will have escaped. Skin flagellates and gill worms, especially, soon abandon the cadaver. Freshly dead fish can be refrigerated without water in a plastic bag for several hours if immediate dissection is not feasible. In this case, even the little water which collects in the plastic bag should be examined for parasites.

2.7. Shipment of Diseased Fish

For many aquarium keepers, the expense of examining fish is too high or they have not as yet mastered this book. There are federal and local government laboratories, however, that might help. Telephone first to ask for packing and shipping instructions. In general, place the fish alone in a plastic bag filled half with air and half with water, then pack that in a well-insulated cardboard box. Ship by air express or by another means if faster in your area.

Shipment in formalin (formaldehyde solution) or in alcohol is irrational, for the internal organs are often already decomposed by the time the fixative has penetrated into them. It is more rational to remove gill arches, spleen, gallbladder, and fragments of the fins, kidney, liver, intestines, and musculature, then pack each separately in a small vial containing the fixative solution described in Chapter 11.8 (E_1). The vials are then packed so they are breakproof and leakproof and shipped. Even like this, many protozoan parasites will hardly still be demonstrable. Send with the specimen all the paperwork that goes with it, including changes in behavior, coloration, and way of swimming, and the last food ingested and quantity. Also describe if any fish died recently, and, if so, how many and at what intervals. Send a water sample when toxicity is suspected.

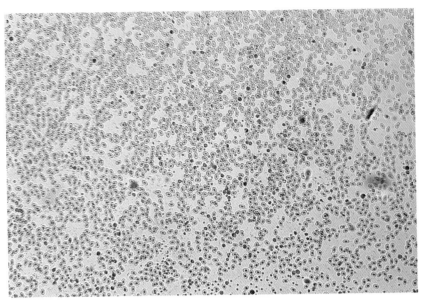

40. Stain E10 makes the nuclei of the blood cells stand out.

enough, otherwise the film will be too thick (Chart 9). The rapidly motile flagellates can be observed at 200 to 400X. Any blood obtained from the excised gill arches can also be examined for flagellates.

To examine the blood cells more closely, add one part methylene blue (Loeffler) to four parts by volume of physiological saline. You can proceed with staining of the slide exactly as described (E_{10}). The cell nucleus of the blood cell slowly stains blue, which can be nicely observed under the microscope (Photograph No. 40). Most of the cells found in the blood are red blood corpuscles (erythrocytes), and only a very few are white blood corpuscles (leukocytes). Fish erythrocytes contain nuclei, but mammalian erythrocytes do not. Unstained mounts do not show the nuclei of the fish erythrocytes or show them only faintly. A successful slide mount shows the erythrocytes lying flat next to one another. Cells standing on edge look like dumbells.

3.4. Gills

The gills will now be thoroughly examined. Cut off the operculum with an opercular incision to lay the gill arches open. The bony gill arches (holobranchia) from which the gill filaments branch off (Photograph No. 4) are exposed (Chart 7). First check the color and condition of the gills and look for parasitic crustaceans. Small, 1-mm-long, white elongated structures that easily come off can be *Ergasilus sieboldi* copepods (Chapter 8.2). Yellowish white modules on the gill filaments are caused by sporozoans (Chapter 6.3). The surface of the gill filaments is enlarged by sickle-shaped gill lamellae in which gaseous exchange occurs. The lamellae are parallel to the gill arches. Their development depends upon the size and kind of fish. Dissect out two gill arches, place one in water on a microscope slide, then dissect several filaments from the other arch, and do the same with them (Chart 10). The first mount is thicker and opaque because the gill arches cannot be squashed flat, but this procedure is still useful because gill worms, which attach themselves only to the bases of the gill filaments, do not show up with the second procedure. The second mount, which is thin enough to look at under high power, can be examined for gill worms, *Oodinium, Ichthyophthirius,* and fungal hyphae.

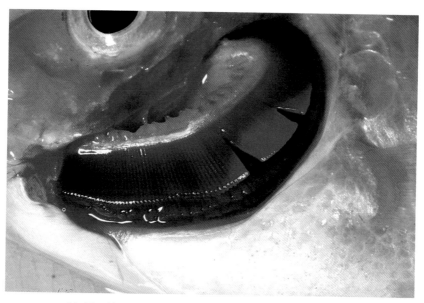

41. Healthy gills are recognized by their bright red color and by their not sticking together.

3.5. Dissection

For dissection or autopsy lay the dead fish in the wax-bottomed tray and stabilize it by pushing a pin through the base of the tail and down into the wax. Do the same through the dorsal musculature. A small pair of sharp-tipped scissors is used to cut open fish that measure less than 10 centimeters (4 in) long. Insert one point of the scissors into the belly just before the anus and cut the belly open, going along between the ventral or the pectoral fins and toward the head (Photograph No. 42). Be careful to cut only along the abdominal wall, not doing any damage to the organs and intestines within the body cavity. This abdominal or ventral incision continues to the gills.

42. Autopsy, showing 1. Ventral incision. 2. Lateral incision. 3. Opercular incision. 4. Cranial incision.

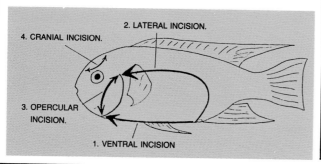

The next cut, the lateral incision, begins at the same place the first (abdominal) incision began, but goes in an arc over the side of the fish and ends at the upper corner of the operculum. Again, be careful not to cut too deeply beyond the body wall, or the air bladder could be torn. The body wall can now be lifted like a flap and laid back over the head, exposing the internal organs (Photograph No. 43).

Adhesions that interfere with lifting the flap of body wall can be teased away carefully with a spatula. If the abdominal wall is too tough to pierce before the anus, then a tip of the scissors can be inserted directly into the anus to begin the incision. In that case, however, be aware that the rectum or colon will be cut, letting intestinal bacteria gain access to the body cavity.

With these incisions, bleeding is normally minimal. The two incisions are connected by a third incision—the opercular incision—running across the operculum to connect the end of the first two incisions, allowing the skin flap to be completely detached. Now the internal organs can be examined for color and condition (Chart 11).

Photographs Nos. 43 and 44 show the approximate positions of the organs. Keep in mind, however, that the size and position of organs may vary from species to species.

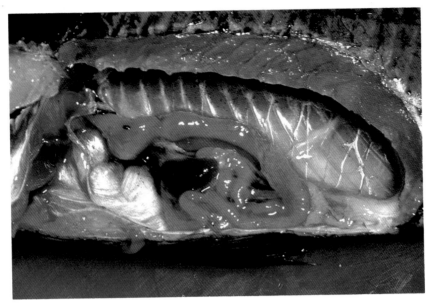

43. Body cavity with organs. Air bladder and liver have
been removed.

Cleanliness is rule number one during the autopsy of fish. To eliminate the chance of transmitting pathogens while working with diseased fish, there must be no eating, drinking, or smoking. Furthermore, take care not to wound yourself with any contaminated instruments. In 1976, Lauer demonstrated that fish tuberculosis bacteria can cause skin lesions in man (but they cannot cause systemic tuberculosis). Wash your hands thoroughly with soap and scrub your fingernails with a nailbrush after the autopsy. Some workers even disinfect their hands with solutions obtained from a

pharmacy or made at home (Chapter 10.2, method D_{50}). Many prefer to wear thin latex gloves during an autopsy.

Removal of the left body wall flap exposes the liver in most fish species (Photographs Nos. 45 and 46). Observe first whether any fluid has collected in the body cavity. Check the gross (i.e., overall) appearance and condition of the visible organs and whether any are bleeding. Prepare a slide of any fluid found in the body cavity, cover with a cover slip, and examine at 200, 400, and 600X, at which magnifications flagellates and blood cells can be easily seen.

44. Position of the organs. Position and shape of the organs can vary from species to species.

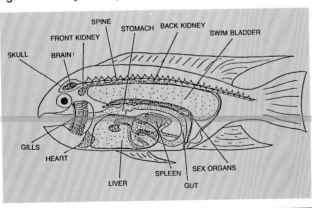

3.6. Liver

A normal liver is usually dark red (Photograph No. 45). The livers of herbivorous fish may appear brownish (Photograph No. 46). A teased specimen of a healthy liver shows a uniformly yellow mass often containing blood vessels (Photograph No. 47). A whitish or milky specimen indicates a pathological fatty condition. Under the microscope, the fat appears as small fluid spheres with dark edges

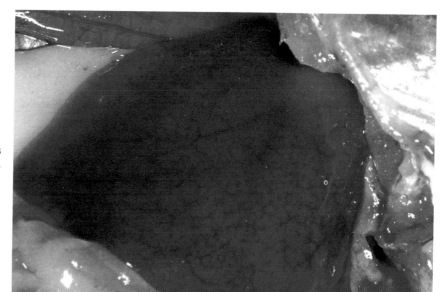

45. The color of a healthy liver is intensely dark red.

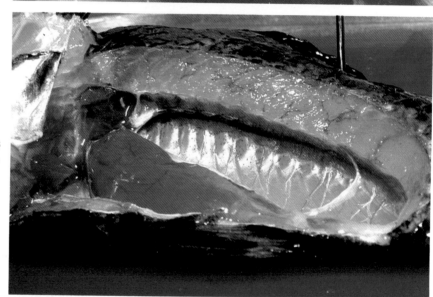

46. The liver of complete vegetarians can be brownish.

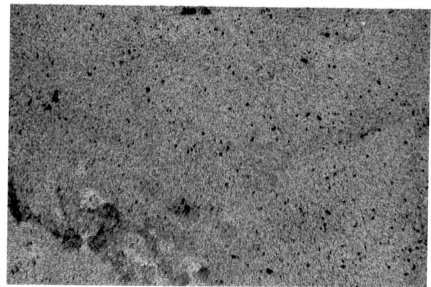

47. Healthy liver of a young discus. Squash mount.

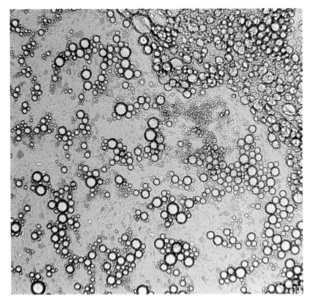

48. Fat droplets expressed by squeezing a fatty liver.

(Photograph No. 48). Examine the slide for flagellates and cysts (such as tuberculosis, *Ichthyophonus,* sporozoans) (Chart 12). A yellow or yellowish brown liver (Photograph No. 49) is not capable of functioning much longer. The cells die off slowly, leading predictably to the fish's death.

49. Severe fatty liver and body cavity.

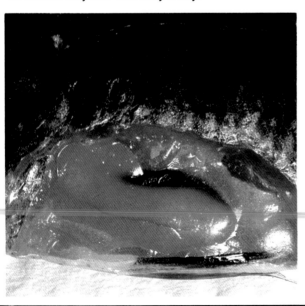

3.7. The Gallbladder

The gallbladder is transparent and filled with green fluid (Photograph No. 50). It is attached to the liver, and its bile duct joins it to the anterior segment of the intestine. Take care in dissecting it out, for its thin wall tears easily, pouring the bile into the body cavity. To prevent that, when removing the gallbladder take it out along with the adjacent pieces of liver and intestine. Once it is on a slide, the gallbladder can be separated from the other organs. If it is damaged there, no great harm is done. Remove the other organ parts and cover with a cover slip. Examine at 100 to 300X for flagellates and worm larvae, and at 600X for bacteria (Chart 13).

3.8. Spleen

The spleen can be seen after pulling apart the intestinal coils. The spleen of many fish is very small, with a color range from dark red to reddish black. The teased specimen under the microscope looks light red, interspersed with lighter circular areas (Photograph No. 51). The scattered yellow brownish clumps of cells are masses of macrophages that remove aging red blood cells from the blood. The spleen is intensely perfused with blood and thus usually is involved first when pathogens enter the bloodstream. Check the tissue for pathologic changes (Chart 15). The surface of the spleen exhibits white nodules when the fish is affected with tuberculosis or *Ichthyophonus.*

3.9. Intestines and Stomach

Particular care is needed whenever dissecting the intestines. The stomach in many species is somewhat thicker than the rest of the intestinal tract and is located anteriorly behind a short esophagus. The stomach is not as distinct in fish as in mammals, and in many fish it is not visibly distinct from the anterior intestines. As an examination specimen, three 1-centimeter lengths are cut, one from the anterior end, one from the middle, and one from the posterior end. The contents of each length are pressed out separately, each in a drop of

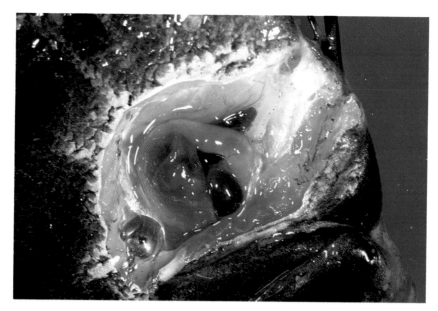

50. The gall bladder is transparent and filled with greenish viscous fluid. In this case, it is pathologically enlarged.

0.64% physiological saline on each of three separate slides (Photograph No. 52). Watch for lesions and cysts in the intestinal wall (Chart 14). Red, bloody areas are inflammations that can be due to improper diet (Photograph No. 29), but can also be due to bacterial infections.

The thin, transparent intestines of smaller fish are placed whole on the slide and teased apart with two dissecting needles to expose the content. Examine at various magnifications to find worms, worm eggs, flagellates, and cysts. Bacteria that are part of the normal intestinal flora usually do not exhibit any movement of their own. Even motile bacteria are rather harmless as long as they do not appear in large numbers.

51. Squash mount of a healthy spleen.

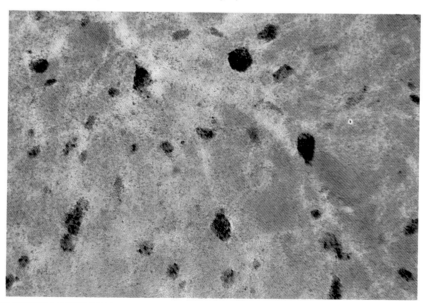

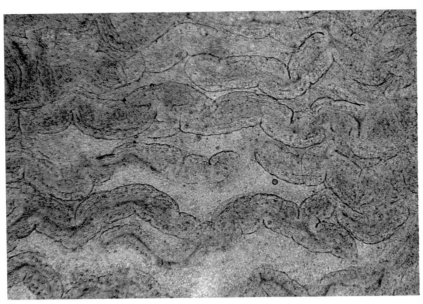

52. Healthy intestines. Folds in the intestinal wall are visible.

3.10. Gonads

Diseases rarely involve the sexual organs. Examine them for fat accumulation and sperm retention. Sporozoan or tubercular cysts are occasionally found in the tissues (Chart 15). The sexual organs are very rarely attacked by nematodes. Injury of the organ tissue during autopsy of male specimens causes release of sperm into the body cavity, finally showing up in slides or other organ tissues and fluids from the body cavity. An inexperienced microscopist can easily mistake the rapidly motile sperm cells for flagellates.

3.11. Air Bladder

In most fish, the air (or gas or swim) bladder is whitish in color and elastic. Check the walls for point hemorrhages and thickened areas (Chart 16). Small, round inclusion bodies in the air bladder wall suggest the presence of *Eimeria* (Chapter 6.3.1), but flagellates and worms can also attack there. In cases of severe inflammation of the air bladder, examination may reveal purulent, bloody fluid. That is often caused by transfer of fish into colder water; even an abrupt drop of 3 to 5°C in temperature is sufficient to cause it. Shifting of abdominal organs in fish that are kept too cold is often caused by an inflammation of the air bladder.

In discus *(Symphysodon)* a new form of air bladder disease has recently been observed. The fish loses some of the gases in the air bladder, so it can no longer stay afloat (that is, in mid-water), but sinks to the bottom and just lies there. The cause is an inflammation of the oval organ or orifice in the anterior ventral area of the air bladder (Photograph No. 30). Passage of gaseous matter through the oval organ into the bloodstream is controlled by a circular muscle (a sphincter). In cases of inflammation this orifice may not close, thus letting the contents of the air bladder escape. In the opposite case, the oval orifice may not open, thus keeping the fish hanging head down just under the surface of the water, where it has to constantly fan with its fins so as not to tip over. Gases are introduced into the air bladder at another place by means of a gas gland called a *rete mirabile,* which is not affected in this disease. Method C_{26} has yielded good therapeutic results.

3.12. Heart

The heart, which often continues to beat long after a fish's death, is examined when there is suspicion of metacercariae, *Ichthyophonus,* or tuberculosis (Chart 15). In such cases, pale nodules are found in the heart wall. In a teased or macerated specimen, small cysts are easily recognized.

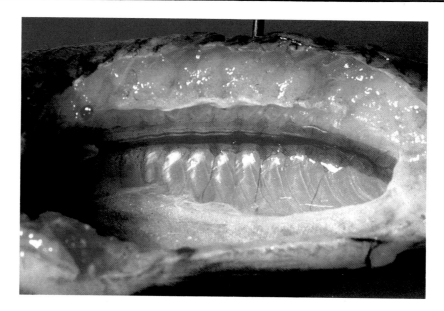

53. In many aquarium fish, the posterior kidney is a narrow strip between the vertebral column and air bladder.

3.13. Kidneys

In bony fish, blood is formed primarily in the kidneys. Therefore, a large number of all types of blood cells are seen in kidney specimens. Generally, the kidney can be reached only after the air bladder is removed (Photograph No. 53). The kidney is differentiated into an anterior or head kidney and a posterior kidney. In smaller fish the posterior kidney often is only a narrow red strip under the vertebral column that thickens anteriorly behind the head, where it forms the head kidney. In many species the head and posterior kidneys are clearly separated from one another. The kidney is blood-red in health, but grayish white when diseased.

Examine the posterior kidney for swellings and cysts of tuberculosis and *Ichthyophonus* (Chart 17). A well-made teased preparation shows, amid the interstitial tissue, the renal tu-

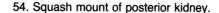

54. Squash mount of posterior kidney.

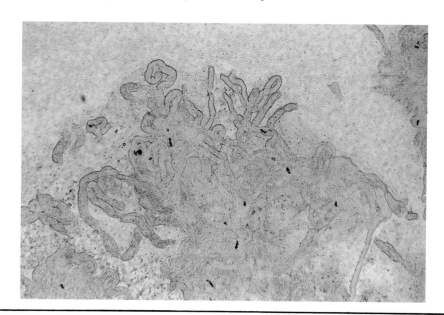

bules (Photograph No. 54), which originate as a thickening containing blood vessels. This thickening is called a Malpighian body (or corpuscle) or a glomerulus. Urine collects there and passes via the uriniferous tubules to the ureter. The constantly beating cilia of the ciliated cells in the Malpighian body flush—really sweep—the urine on its way. These cilia can be seen only in well-made slides and should not be confused with bacteria. The interstitial tissue looks yellow to yellow-brown and contains many blood capillaries and lymphocytes.

3.14. Brain

The brain rarely becomes diseased, but tuberculosis and *Ichthyophonus* cysts are often found in it. It is exposed by a skull or cranial incision (Chart 18). Take a small sample of the white mass and tease it apart in the usual manner on a glass slide. Under the microscope, the specimen is a uniformly white mass interspersed with small, irregular blood vessel (Photograph No. 55).

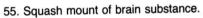

55. Squash mount of brain substance.

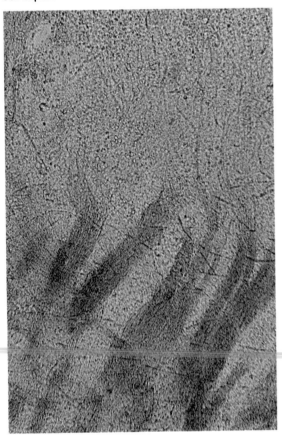

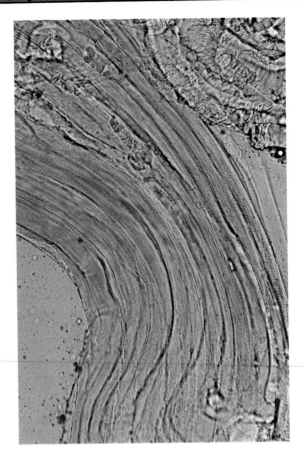

56. Squash mount of muscle.

3.1.5. Musculature

Muscles consist of adjacent but not connected muscle fibers and connective tissue. Samples are cut from the flank of the dorsal musculature and teased out to prepare a slide (Photograph No. 56). Examine the slide for cestode (tapeworm) and nematode (roundworm) larvae, as well as for sporozoa, mycobacteria, and *Ichthyophonus* (Chart 18). Cysts of many kinds of bacteria destroy the tissue, causing large lesions in the muscles. Dissect away the lesion so it is not confused with a sporozoan cyst. Then tease apart a sample of it for mounting on a slide. Prepare fresh mounts of the fluid contents in order to see whether motile or immotile bacteria are present. Stain thin smears or squash mounts according to methods E_7 and E_8.

Chapter 4
Viral and Bacterial Diseases

4.1. Purely Viral Diseases

The word *virus*—Latin for *slime, juice,* or *poison*—was for a long time the general name for any kind of pathogen. Today the name virus is restricted to pathogenic particles that are so small that they pass through filters that hold bacteria. Viruses live on borrowed life, for they are too small to maintain any metabolism of their own. They consist only of a chemical shell that contains a genetic molecule (RNA). If the virus touches a cell, it attaches itself firmly to the wall and injects its RNA into the cell. The viral RNA then takes over the cellular metabolism, forcing it to produce new viruses, which often destroy the cell.

Viruses are too small to see with an optical microscope, so their presence can be confirmed only in institutions with the proper facilities. Viruses are usually recognized along with the symptomatology of each disease they cause. Lymphocystis is certainly the best known viral fish disease (Photograph No. 15, Chart 5). This disease often appears first on the fins, but then spreads over the whole body, eventually killing the fish. Lymphocystis infections can easily be seen with the naked eye, since the virus causes the skin cells to grow abnormally large (Photograph No. 57). The often whitish clumps of cells commonly resemble small clutches of eggs adhering to the skin, but sometimes only a few cells may appear over the whole area of the body. The skin feels rough when stroked. Internal organs are rarely affected. Lymphocystis is transmitted predominantly via the contents of burst cells. The behavior of any fish affected by it does not reveal any adverse effects. Treatment can be successful when the disease is recognized early enough. Upon early recognition, cut the affected part out of the fin and isolate the victim under optimal conditions. Continue to treat any open wounds like injuries (Chapter 10, method A_4 or C_1). It is more humane to painlessly put severely affected fish out of their misery and destroy them. Fish which appear to be otherwise healthy must be observed 60 days in quarantine. When frequent outbreaks occur, quarantine the remaining healthy fish and disinfect the aquarium according to method D_1, D_3, or D_5 (Chapter 10.2).

The throat swellings often observed in black mollies have also been ascribed to the effect of viruses (Schaeperclaus, 1954). They are difficult to differentiate from thryoid swellings (Chapter 9.1). Other diseases, too, are possibly caused by viruses. Viral diseases that occur in economically useful fish possibly also occur in similar or somewhat different forms in aquarium fish. Since this is still a little-explored area, it is possible that diseases of unknown origin may be caused by viruses.

57. Squash mounted cells affected with *Lymphocystis.* Size: 120-250u.

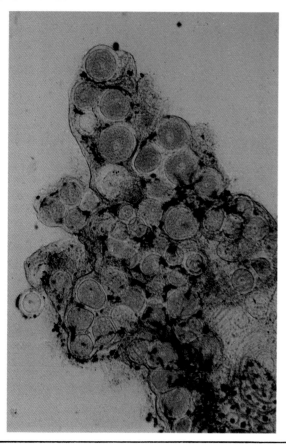

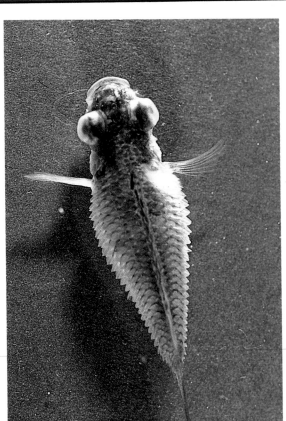

58. Scales lifted up and popeyes in abdominal dropsy.

4.2. Abdominal Dropsy

Infectious abdominal dropsy has been extensively studied in carp. Obviously, not all experience from economic fish can be applied to aquarium fish, but there are parallels when aquarium fish are affected (Photograph No.58). Viruses indeed infect the fish, but bacteria are always involved, so that at times they are seen as the primary cause. In aquarium fish, it still has not been established whether the signs are caused primarily by viruses or whether a purely bacterial infection is involved. Almost all fish species can be affected. Even without a specific host, the bacteria can remain viable and reproduce for months in the water and mud. Since they belong to the normal bacterial flora of the tank, healthy fish can resist them. The fish are endangered only when starvation, improper diet, cold, or transportation stresses them, or when unsanitary conditions in the tank burden them.

Once a fish is infected, it releases large numbers of bacteria, exposing its tankmates to the disease, which is often characterized by the discharge of large amounts of fluid into the body cavity. In many cases, the belly of the fish looks as if it were bloated to the bursting point. Skin lesions, too, can appear, as well as small vesicles along the lateral line (Photograph No. 14, Chart 5). The fish often rock back and forth just under the surface of the water and lack their flight reflex or else exhibit it only to a very limited extent. The ocular reflex also is weaker. The anus is often inflamed and sometimes puffed out. Fins clamp together. If an affected kidney reaches the advanced stage, then anemia causes the gills to become pale. Usually pop-eye (exophthalmos) also occurs. Intestinal mucosa sloughs off and is eliminated, so dissection reveals a transparent, glassy intestinal wall. The fluid in the body cavity is clear, but often yellowish or bloody. It can be fully liquid or viscous in consistency (Photograph No. 24, Chart 11). The kidney is inflamed, the liver yellow to light brown, and the cells slough off. Sometimes many fat droplets are seen in a squash preparation. The gallbladder is often very swollen, its contents dark green. Many motile and immotile bacteria are found in the liver, gallbladder, kidney, and body cavity. Skeletal deformations often cause spinal curvature. Treatment is possible during the early stage. Affected fish and those suspected of the disease immediately should be isolated and observed.

Abdominal dropsy of aquarium fish does not involve any specific symptomatology. The above-described symptoms can appear simultaneously or separately. It is also possible that the fish become emaciated or die without any outward signs. Any bacteria found usually belong to just a few genera. As a rule, however, motile and immotile Gram-negative rods measuring 1 to 3 microns are found in the fluid from the body cavity, as well as in the liver, spleen, and kidney. Diagnosis requires staining with the Ziehl/Neelsen stain (Chapter 11, method E_8) to eliminate the possibility of tuberculosis. Then a specimen is prepared with Gram's stain (Chapter 11, method E_7).

For treatment, methods C_{25}, A_5, A_6, and A_1 are suitable. Method C_{21} may be useful in the initial stage of the disease. Method C_{21} is the treatment of choice for prophylactic treatment of the other fish from the same tank. Following an epidemic of abdominal dropsy, the aquarium and its contents must be thoroughly disinfected according to methods D_1, D_3, or D_5 (Chapter 10.2). The most appropriate hygienic conditions must be instituted as prophylaxis. Fish whose livers or kidneys are too badly damaged will die after a while despite any treatment.

4.3. Furunculosis

Furunculosis infections have been recognized in the Salmonidae (trouts and salmons) since the turn of the century. They are caused by bacteria of the genus *Aeromonas,* particularly *Aeromonas salmonicida.* It forms purulent boils and lesions measuring 2 to 20 mm. The fins become inflamed and frayed. Sometimes only turbidity—either slight or severe—shows on the fins. Fungal overgrowth often occurs as a secondary infection.

A second type of symptomatology involves small hemorrhages in the internal organs, skin, gills, fins, and musculature. The pathogens are transmitted when the fish ingest fecal matter on the cadavers of infected fish and also via skin parasites. Transmission is also possible when purulent matter from ruptured lesions enters the water. Poor water quality fosters spread of the disease. Thorough disinfection of the aquarium is required. If relapse occurs several weeks after successful treatment, poor hygienic conditions in the tank may be the cause. The pathogens are short, Gram-negative, immotile rod-shaped bacteria measuring 1.7 to 2 microns. The rods often occur in pairs and chains. Treatment can be started with method C_{25}. If no improvement occurs, resort to method A_5 or A_1. Fish that do not exhibit any symptoms can be treated prophylactically with method C_{21}.

4.4. Fin Rot

Bacterial fin rot is a widely occurring disease that mainly affects younger fish. The disease begins with turbidity of the fin margins, which finally turn white. The tissue between the fin rays breaks apart so that the fins fray and rot away (Photograph No. 16, Chart 6). The bases of the fins become inflamed and red. The inner organs are not affected. After removal of the cause and drug treatment, regrowth of the fins is possible.

Smears of fin remnants show large quantities of motile, Gram-negative, rod-shaped bacteria. In rare cases, fungus covers the damaged areas. The pathogens belong to the genera *Aeromonas, Pseudomonas,* and *Vibrio. Aeromonas* bacteria measure between 1 and 2.2 microns, *Pseudomonas* between 1 and 2.5 microns, and *Vibrio* about 1.5 microns. Treatment consists of method C_1, C_{21}, or C_3. Methods A_3 and A_1 also are very effective.

Bacterial fin rot occurs because of poor maintenance or as a result of another disease. Good water quality is a preventive. Oxygen depletion, water contaminated with fecal matter, too high a pH value, and dissolved heavy metals can encourage the disease. Treatment is successful only when the source is found and removed. In the early stage, transfer of the fish to clean water is often enough, and the fins regrow.

4.5. *Vibrio* Infections

The symptomatology of *Vibrio* infections has been recognized for 200 years. It was from North Sea eels at the beginning of this century that bacteria of the species *Vibrio anguillarum* were first isolated and identified. Since then it has become known that *Vibrio* infections occur worldwide, predominantly in marine and brackish water fish as well as shrimps. In isolated instances this pathogen has been found in freshwater fish. In marine fish the disease often follows only a latent course. In sensitive fish whose power of resistance has been weakened, the disease is expressed through convulsive twitching and death. The fish may not even show any other outward signs. Spleenic and renal swelling as well as severe hemorrhaging in the body cavity and skin often occur. Resistant fish, however, often show only minor hemorrhages and intestinal inflammations. Fish in all temperature zones are susceptible. The pathogens can be found in any affected organs.

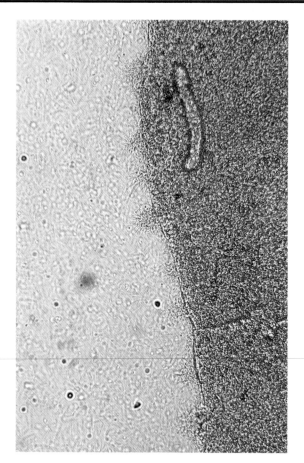

59. *Columnaris* bacteria form small heaps (30-35 u) at the edges of scales and fins. Bright—field photgraph. (400X).

Vibrio anguillarum is a Gram-negative, very motile flagellated bacterium. These slightly curved cells measure between 0.4 to 0.6 microns x 1.2 to 2 microns. The flagellum is 4 to 6 microns long. The cells often form chains, which makes them seem longer. Aquarium fish seldom exhibit a pure *Vibrio* infection, especially in long-lasting courses, when large amounts of *Pseudomonas, Aeromonas,* and cocci can be found in the various organs.

The disease is favored by high temperatures, overcrowded tanks, stress, noxious substances in the water, and poor water quality. Treatment by methods A_5, A_6, and A_1 is usually, but not always, successful.

4.6. Columnaris Disease

The cause of this relatively frequent disease in the aquarium is the bacterium *Flexibacter columnaris.* At first it forms small whitish spots on the snout, on the edges of the scales, and on the fins, which when larger give the impressions of mold (Photograph No. 12, Chart 5). The fin edges begin to disintegrate, leaving the fin rays bare. The affected areas of skin often become covered with fungus. The gills also can be affected, the gill filaments disintegrating from the tip to the gill arch. In young fish the filaments stick together because of extreme swelling of the gill epithelium and considerable mucus or slime secretion. The supply of oxygen is blocked and rapid breathing is the result. This condition often is called bacterial gill disease or bacterial gill rot.

A smear of material from the affected side of the body is taken for diagnosis or a tiny specimen can be cut from the fin margins. At higher power can be seen bacteria up to 8 microns long and 0.7 microns wide that glide along slowly but do not possess any flagella (Photograph No. 60). After a short while, some break away and collect under the cover slip, where many of the columnaris bacteria oscillate with their free ends. They also clump together as columns or piles at the margin of the inflamed tissue areas (Photograph No. 59).

There are two distinct forms of columnaris disease. During the chronic course, the white areas very gradually enlarge and the fish die many days later. In the acute form, the white spots spread out visibly within several hours. A population of more than 100 fish may all die within three days, so treatment must be instituted quickly. Higher water temperatures accelerate the course of the disease. Points of attack for columnaris infections are skin wounds as well as epithelial damage occasioned by vitamin deficiency. Poor water quality, high ammonia concentration, and low oxygen content all contribute.

Treatment is possible but is only successful over a long period when optimal maintenance conditions have been established. Various methods have been used for the chronic and acute forms. The chronic form can be treated with method C_{1c}, C_{1d}, or A_1. Since there is no time for a test in the acute form, method A_2 is applied at once. With methods E_7 and E_9, the bacteria can be stained to differentiate them.

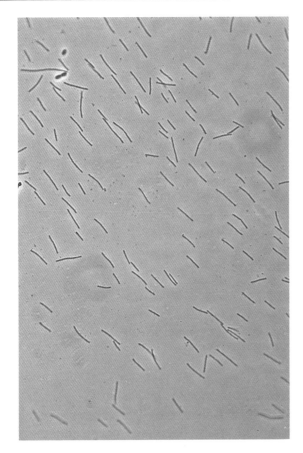

60. Single *columnaris* bacterium. Phase contrast photograph. Bacterial length: 5-8u.

4.7. Piscine Tuberculosis

As in man, tuberculosis in fish is also caused by mycobacteria. It breaks out mainly during weakened states of health, poor living conditions, and vitamin deficiencies. Fish in heavily populated aquariums are particularly at risk. Mycobacteria occur everywhere, but mostly in the bottom soil, debris, food remnants, and dead fish. The disease often runs a lingering course, with some fish dying now and then over several months. At other times it strikes as an epidemic and within a few weeks kills the whole population.

The external indications of a tubercular infection vary from species to species and from one individual to another, depending upon their varying degrees of resistance. Additionally, the symptoms also show up in other diseases, so they are a danger signal only when verified at autopsy. Symptoms could include: bloating of the body caused by fluid accumulation in the body cavity; emaciation along the narrow dorsal ridge (razorback) and sunken belly; scale loss and lifted scales; open skin lesions (Photograph No. 4, Chart 3); pop-eye to the point of the eyes actually popping out; spinal curvature; pale coloration; jerky swimming; abdominal organ displacement; greatly reduced reactions and reflexes; loss of appetite; and remaining apart from other fish ("standing in the corner"). These symptoms can appear alone or in various combinations.

After autopsy, specimens are teased apart to prepare a slide mount. In severe infections, examination with a hand lens reveals whitish gray nodules on the liver and spleen as a defensive reaction of the organism, which is attempting to surround the bacterial foci of infection with connective tissue to isolate them from healthy tissue. Examination under the microscope reveals a uniformly yellowish to light brown content of the cysts because the con-

61. Tubercular cysts in squash mount. Cyst diameter between 180 and 300u.

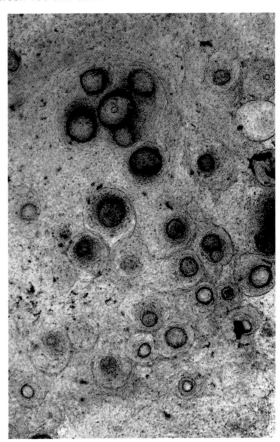

nective tissue capsule is translucent and colorless. The cysts easily can be confused with *Ichthyophonus* (see the next chapter). In contrast to these, the tubercular cysts are not always round. In a pronounced *Mycobacterium* infection, you can usually find round, elongated, and branched cysts in a squash preparation (Photograph No. 61). Confusion with *Ichthyophonus* is not a great problem because neither condition can be treated. Differentiation, however, is possible by staining the squashed cysts according to method E_8, Chapter 11, revealing red-stained 1 to 5 microns x 0.2 to 0.6 micron rod-shaped bacteria (Photograph No. 119, Chapter 11.8.7). These organisms are immotile when alive.

Tubercular cysts often also are found in the organs of fish that were autopsied due to death from other diseases. Tubercular cysts can rupture when environmental conditions deteriorate or the fish are overstressed. Then the mycobacteria spread out in the fish and attack other organs. As countermeasures, the best quality conditions (diet, water, temperature, etc.) possible are recommended. Quarantine any visibly ill fish and also those suspected of being diseased. Once tuberculosis is verified, the diseased fish must be sacrificed and destroyed. When a whole tank is struck with an epidemic, sacrifice all the fish and then thoroughly disinfect the tank and all equipment according to method D_1, D_3, or D_5 (Chapter 10).

Chapter 5
FUNGAL AND ALGAL DISEASES

5.1. External Mycoses

Fungi are present in every aquarium. They normally are among the invisible helpers that break down food remnants and fecal matter in the filter and in inaccessible spots in the tank. Fungal spores float around in the water until they land upon suitable material upon which to germinate. They do not care for healthy skin of the fish. Only if the integrity of the skin is damaged by bites or other wounds can the spores penetrate it and germinate. Bacterial infections and skin parasites also can be the precipitating factors in fungal diseases. Prophylactic measures can be effective against fungal infections. Once a mycotic disease becomes so established, however, that the filaments (hyphae) show up clearly at the injured site, any help usually comes too late (Photograph No. 11, Chart 5). The pathogens are fungi of the genera *Saprolegnia, Achlya,* and *Dictyuchus.* They normally live on dead organic matter such as food remnants and the remains of dead food animals. Fungus also attacks dead eggs. The eggs turn white because the egg-white coagulates, not because of the fungus. Only in a later stage do the fungal filaments visibly grow on the white eggs. If there are too many dead eggs in one clutch, then the growing fungus also may spread to and attack the healthy eggs.

Fungal infections caused by the above genera show up as thin white threads (the hyphae) at the infected spots, building up their mass until they look like puffs of raw cotton that are visible to the naked eye. For microscopic examination, snip off a cottony puff of filaments and prepare a slide mount. Even at low power the fungal filaments and the spore-filled sporangia at their tips are visible (Photograph No. 62). Heavily infected fish usually cannot be saved, because the fungal filaments also grow into the fish and do severe damage to the organs. Besides, they usually release toxic metabolic products that adversely affect the fish. The cause of the infection should be found and cleared up before treatment starts.

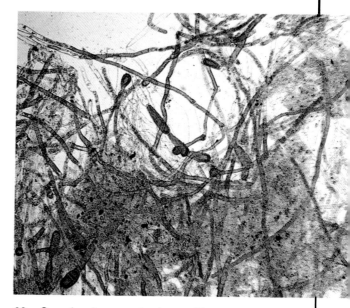

62. *Saprolegnia* spp. hyphae with spore capsules. Length of meshed spore capsules in the middle of the picture: 440u.

Fungi can be controlled by bathing the fish in various medicated solutions. The choice of the medication depends upon the severity of the infestation. Methods C_{12} and C_{17} can be used for prophylaxis and for mild infestation. As prophylaxis against fungal attack on eggs, method C_{17e} for three days is effective. Methods C_{23} and C_9 can be used for fungal involvement of wounds and also large areas.

5.2. Internal Mycoses

5.2.1. *Ichthyophonus hoferi (Ichthyosporidium)*

Ichthyophonus hoferi (formerly called *Ichthyosporidium*) was some years ago one of the most dreaded organisms in the aquarium. Today the thought is that tuberculosis bacteria are the culprit in most cases, since it is very difficult to distinguish them from *Ichthyophonus.* The disease occurs in both marine and freshwater fish. The whole population of the tank can be at risk if the fish are weakened and kept in unhygienic aquariums. The opinion that *Ichthyophonus* cannot occur in tropical aquarium fish because of the high temperature has been refuted. Dr.H. Herkner demonstrated in 1961 that feeding diseased marine fish to tropical fish elicited the disease in 20% of the latter.

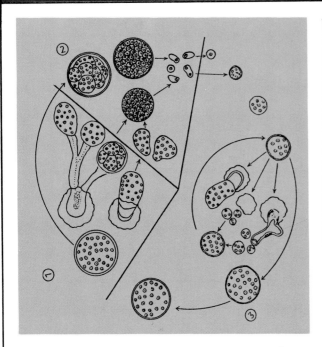

63. *Ichthyophonus hoferi.* The Development Cycle. Drawn after Dorier and Degrange. Taken from Reichenbach-Klinke's *Krankheiten und Schädignun der Fische.*

1. The white cysts are roundish to elliptical. The fish become infected by eating infective plasmodia with their food. 2. The digestive juice "hatches" the plasmodia into amoeboid embryos which are mostly excreted. 3. The ones which are not excreted enter the bloodstream and are distributed in organs throughout the fish's body.

The name of the pathogen is *Ichthyophonus hoferi,* classified under the Phycomycetes. Up to recently it was called *Ichthyosporidium hoferi,* but based on recent studies the name was changed (Reichenbach-Klinke, 1980). The discoverer of the disease, B. Hofer, called it the tumbling disease (Taumelkrankheit in German) because affected fish rocked or swayed as they swam. Otherwise, there is usually nothing external to see, except sometimes skin lesions in the Anabantidae and holes in the heads of cichlids (false hole disease). The organs preferentially affected are liver, spleen, heart, kidney, and brain. The gonads, gills, and musculature are not affected as often.

Fish thought to harbor *Ichthyophonus* are sacrificed and autopsied. The white cysts on the organs are generally visible without any special preparation. For diagnosis, prepare teased specimens of liver, heart, spleen, and kidney, and examine them at 50 to 100X. The 0.04 to 2 mm cysts are easy to find in the slide mount. They are roundish to elliptical in shape,

look brown with black particles inside, and are enveloped in pale connective tissue. Squash preparations stained according to method E_8 (Chapter 11.8) do not show any bacteria.

The fish become infected by ingesting infective plasmodia with their food. The effect of the digestive juices breaks these plasmodia up into amoeboid embryos, most of which are eliminated. The few remaining ones are capable of penetrating the intestinal wall and letting themselves be carried by the bloodstream to the organs. That is more apt to happen in a weakened fish because the intestines of healthy fish are more resistant. A varied, healthy diet is an important preventive measure. The parasite grows in the infected organ by repeated nuclear divisions then encapsulates itself for a resting phase of several days. Since the fish, too, encapsulates the parasite, confusion with tuberculosis is easily possible at this stage (Photograph No. 63). Multinuclear plasmodia hatch from the cysts and divide into daughter cells, which then infiltrate the organs. The fish dies if the affected organs can no longer function. After the death of the host fish, hyphae grow out of the cysts and give rise to the infective plasmodia at their tips. Transmission occurs when the dead fish are eaten. All freshwater and marine fish appear to be susceptible to the disease (Reichenback-Klinke). No treatment is known. Dead fish must be removed from the aquarium and destroyed.

5.2.2. *Aphanomyces*

Besides *Ichthyophonus,* other fungi have been discovered that penetrate fish organs by means of their mycelia. External signs are often lacking, except that the reactions and movements of the affected animals are inhibited. Tropical freshwater fish are said to occasionally exhibit an epidemic-like response to infection with *Aphanomyces* species. This fungus grows in the dorsal musculature. Death ensues in several days when the skin is broken through from inside. Teased specimens of the organ tissues can be stained to better define the fungal hyphae. Since these mycoses seldom occur in the aquarium, no more need be said of them.

5.2.3. *Branchiomyces,* Gill Rot

This gill mycosis occurs most frequently in fish that live in water severely burdened with organic pollution. The pathogen can be introduced into the aquarium via live food. Gill rot is not a danger in clean aquariums in which the water is changed regularly. It is a danger, however, in garden ponds with heavy algal growth during the warm season. The causes are fungi of the genus *Branchiomyces.* They grow in gill epithelium, infiltrate the tissue, and obstruct circulation. The affected gill filaments die, decompose, and fall off (Photograph No. 18, Chart 7). The fish become lethargic, gasp for air, breathe with difficulty, and finally suffocate. For examination, tease off several of the dead gill filaments and prepare a mount. The fungal hyphae can be recognized at 100X (Photgraph No. 64). Treatment by methods C_{12}, C_3, and C_9 is possible.

64. *Branchiomyces* spp. infection of gills

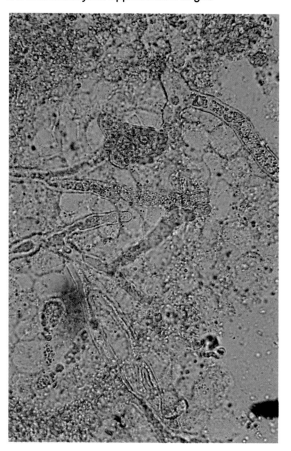

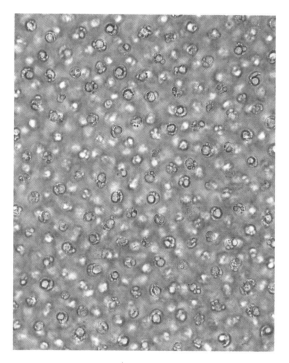

65. *Dermocystidium* spores from cysts shown in Table 6, picture 17. Spore size 5u.

5.3. Algal Diseases

In general, algae do not threaten aquarium fish. There are, however, algae that secrete toxic substances that may endanger the fish. For that, however, intensive reproduction and heavy growth are required. Additionally, the probability of introducing a toxic algal species is very slight. Many green algal species grow on opercula and fins but do not cause any damage as long as their growth is controlled. A quick bath, such as in C_{17c}, helps.

5.4. *Dermocystidium*

It is still undecided how to classify *Dermocystidium*. Many authors assign it to the fungi, but others put it with the Haplospora. *Dermocystidium* forms cysts in the skin and gills (Photograph No. 17, Chart 6). The cysts can be either round or elongated and almost worm-like, measuring 1 to 10 mm or more. The cyst is filled with a hundred thousand tiny spores, each measuring 3 to 6 microns. The spores are round and reveal several round structures of various sizes inside (Photograph No. 65). There is no known treatment.

Chapter 6
PATHOGENIC PROTOZOA

6.1. Flagellates

Protozoa are all one-celled organisms that consist of a cell nucleus enclosed by a cell membrane. They include a whole array of species that parasitize fish. Many of them cause fatal diseases if the fish are not treated in time.

Flagellates are very small but can be recognized at 100X and up because of their motility. To identify them, however, requires 600X and keen observation of their mode of swimming or fixation by staining (Chapter 11.8.4, method E_6). They move by means of one or more whip-like organs (flagella). They reproduce by

66. *Trypanosoma* spp. and *Cryptobia* spp. with red blood cells. Scale 10u. Size: 10-25u. From Amiacher, Doflein and Timofeev, as well as my own observations.

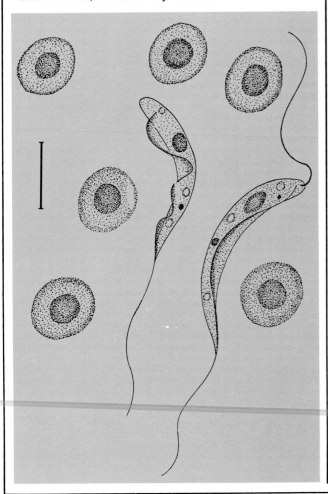

longitudinal division (fission). Flagellates occur on the skin, in the intestine, in the internal organs, and in the blood of fish. It is possible that a specific flagellate genus that is highly pathogenic for one fish species will not affect another fish species.

6.1.1. Blood Flagellates

The most widely known blood flagellates are species of the genera *Cryptobia* and *Trypanosoma* (Photograph No. 66). They measure 10 to 25 microns in length and thus are somewhat larger than blood cells. Their rapid movement makes them easy to recognize in a blood smear (Chapter 3.3). Freshwater and marine fish can be affected.

Cryptobia is a flagellate with two flagella. In a severe infection the fish become lethargic, with greatly reduced reactions and reflexes. In advanced cases the fish can be caught by hand, which is why the term "fish sleeping sickness" is sometimes used. The mode of swimming is unnatural: many fish rotate about their horizontal axis or swim head down. They become emaciated and their gills turn pale.

Transmission to other fish occurs via blood-sucking parasites such as, for example, flukes and leeches. Since these normally are not in an aquarium, transmission to healthy fish is hardly a danger. Blood parasites are not rare in pond fish, so care must be taken not to introduce into the aquarium any flukes or leeches along with live foods. Fish captured in the wild as well as goldfish are often affected with blood flagellates. The pathogens are identified either directly in the blood (Chapter 3.3) or in a teased specimen from the kidney. Treatment with methylene blue can be tried for a week (Chapter 10, method C_{17} or C_{17b}).

Trypanosoma is hardly distinguishable from *Cryptobia* (Photograph No. 66). At high power with a good microscope or with phase contrast illumination, *Trypanosoma* can be seen to have only one flagellum. Infestation with them is harmless, since these single-flagellum flagellates do not damage the fish.

6.1.2. Intestinal Flagellates

Intestinal flagellates can be found in many fish to which they do no harm. The pathogenicity of the organisms varies from fish to fish; thus angelfish may not be affected at all by the same flagellates that damage discus. The best known genera of intestinal flagellates are *Hexamita, Spironucleus, Trichomonas,* and *Bodomonas.*

Hexamita and *Bodomonas* are difficult to identify (Photographs Nos. 67 and 70). *Hexamita,* which used to be called *Octomitus,* attacks the intestines, gallbladder, and also is sometimes found in the blood. Fish affected by intestinal flagellates isolate themselves from the others, become emaciated, excrete white and slimy feces, darken their coloration, and often swim backward (Photograph No. 2, Chart 3). Many fish exhibit a swollen body. We do not yet know the extent to which these flagellates damage marine fish in aquariums. Marine fish in the wild do not seem to be affected by them. *Hexamita* infections are rare in ornamental fish; any similar infection usually is due to *Spironucleus.* Neither is the "hole disease" in cichlids, especially the discus, caused by *Hexamita.* According to Dr. Schubert, *Hexamita* has never been found in discus. Even the *Spironucleus* flagellate is only one of the possible causes of "hole disease" in cichlids (Chapter 9.3). The intestines are most affected can contain millions of these flagellates. Spread to the gallbladder and blood is possible, in which case the infection usually runs a fatal course.

Fresh fecal matter excreted from the living fish is prepared for examination. Specimens from fish that just died or were just sacrificed should include fragments of the rectum, colon, and gallbladder. Examination is according to guidelines in Chapter 3.9. Identification of the genus can only be made from fixed specimens (described in Chapter 11.8.4, method E$_6$). The flagellates can be seen at 120X up; identification requires 300 to 400X

Hexamita and *Spironucleus* possess an elongated, oval cell. Of the eight anterior flagella, two trail rearward along a groove on the surface of the cell. Posteriorly they trail well beyond the end of the cell. The six remaining anterior flagella are very motile and provide locomotion (Photographs Nos. 67, 68 and 71). Both flagellates swim jerkily in a straight line, with *Hexamita* somewhat slower than *Spironucleus. Hexamita salmonis* measures 8 to 12 microns in length by 6 to 8 microns across. *Spironucleus elegans* is slightly shorter—8 to 11 microns long by 4 to 6 microns thick. *Spironucleus* nuclei are larger than those of *Hexamita.*

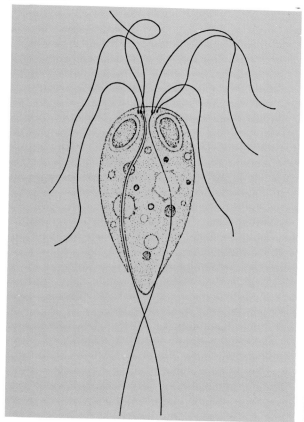

67. *Hexamita* spp. Size: 7-12u. From Kulda and Lom, as well as my own observations.

Trichomonids have sack-shaped cells with an average length of 12 microns (Photograph No. 72). From the upper pole originate four flagella, three of which beat up and down in the water. The fourth flagellum undulates from top to bottom along the cell surface, with which it is connected by a thin membrane (the undulating membrane). Trichomonids swim very slowly, rolling lethargically along. The techniques of fixing specimens to render the flagella recognizable are given in Chapter 11.8.4, method E$_6$.

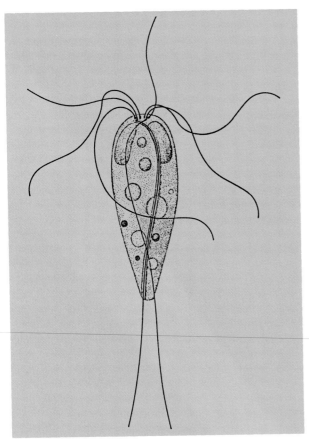

68. *Spironucleus* spp. Size 10-14u. From Kulda and Lom, as well as my own observations.

Flagellates of the genus *Bodomonas* possess a spindle-shaped, streamlined cell with two flagella at the anterior end. One is directed rearward and lies against the cell body but is not connected with the cell membrane (Photographs Nos. 69 and 70). The second flagellum is freely motile. At the anterior end, that is, the pole facing the direction of flagellation, a large bright spot, not the nucleus, can be recognized at 800 to 1000X. It appears to be an organelle of attachment because in well-made mounts of the intestinal wall innumerable flagellates can be observed as they attach themselves with this organelle to the cell wall and beat their flagella around in the intestinal lumen. Since the flagellates hang in large numbers and in the same direction, the intestinal mucosa at these places looks, under about 200X, like a wind-blown meadow. These still unidentified flagellates measure 10 to 14 microns. Their movement is rapid, undulating, and gyrating.

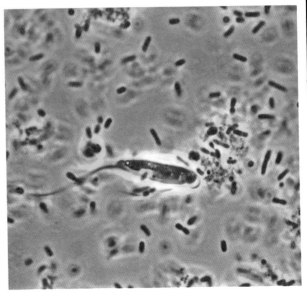

69. *Bodomonas* spp. Scale: 16u.

Heavy losses among mainly Malawi cichlids have been caused in recent years by a *Cryptobia* species that parasitizes exclusively the intestine. The affected fish discharge white feces and die within a few days, their bellies bloated. The parasite's mode of locomotion is not distinguishable from *Bodomonas* spp., but it attains 16 to 24 microns in size. The trailing flagellum is connected to the surface of the cell body by means of a narrow undulating membrane.

Method C_{19} or Hex-Ex can be used to treat for *Hexamita, Spironucleus,* and *Trichomonas.* These methods, however, don't work for *Bodomonas* and *Cryptobia;* only method C_8 can be used against these two genera.

6.1.3. Skin Flagellates
The flagellates that parasitize fish skin can severely damage their host, since skin is a vi-

70. *Bodomonas* spp. Scale: 10u.

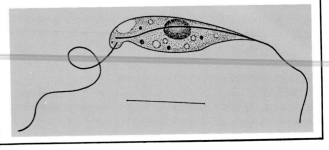

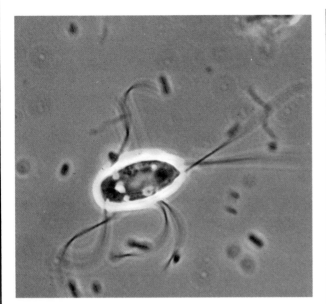

71. *Spironucleus* spp. Size: 12u. (Phase contrast photograph).

tal organ (Chapter 3.2). Aquarium hobbyists are very familiar with *Costia necatrix* (formerly *Ichthyobodo),* a small bean-shaped (reniform) organism, and also with various species of the dinoflagellate genus *Oodinium.*

6.1.3.1. *Costia necatrix*

Costia necatrix is a small flagellate measuring 8 to 12 microns. Two flagella originate at the anterior pole of the cell. In a smear *Costia* looks bean-shaped, but when attached to the skin it takes on a pear shape (Photograph No. 73). With its thin end it attaches itself tightly to the skin and destroys it. In a moderately severe infection the mucosa appears turbid; severe infection can lead to disintegration of the skin and bleeding (Photograph No. 10, Chart 5). There usually are other flagellates and ciliates also at the affected skin sites, but these are not real parasites (Chapters 6.4.5 and 6.4.6). Fungal overgrowth can occur as a result. *Costia* is a parasite upon weakness, for healthy adult fish can resist infection. Young fish, however, are more susceptible.

Marine fish can be somewhat affected if *Costia* is introduced along with food fish into saltwater aquariums, but the parasites then generally are not pathogenic.

Skin and gill smears are used in diagnosis. The tumbling *Costia* can be seen at a magnifi-

cation of at least 300X. They often somersault or spring over short distances, sometimes suddenly disappearing from the field then reappearing in a fraction of a second quite some distance away.

Costia necatrix can survive only on fish. Without a host it perishes in an hour, contracting into a sphere. *Costia* cannot tolerate temperatures over 30°C, so there is the possibility of controlling it by raising the temperature to 32°C (Chapter 10, method B_1). As a preventive against infections, add methylene blue to the water (Chapter 10, method C_{17}). Effective chemical treatments include methods C_3, C_{13}, and C_{1c}. Method C_7, however, can be used only on unbroken skin in the early stage. For prevention and with incipient infections, treatment can be according to methods C_{12} and C_{17}.

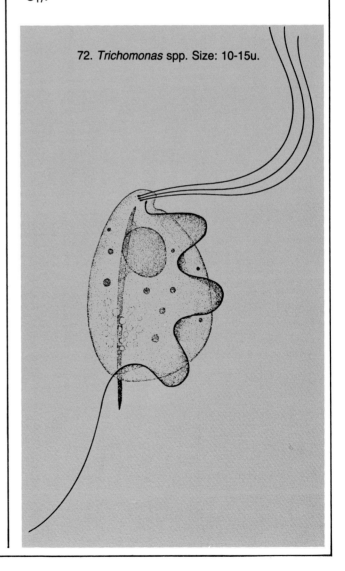

72. *Trichomonas* spp. Size: 10-15u.

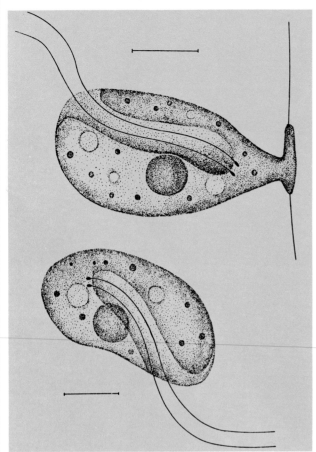

73. *Costia necatrix.* Size: 10-15u. Scale 3 u. From Jojon and Lom, as well as my own observations.

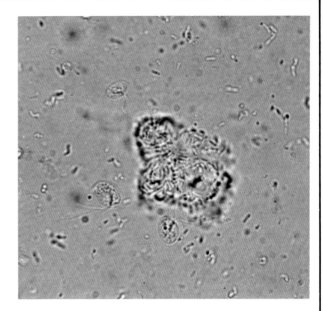

74. Two specimens of *Costia* spp. in a skin smear. Size: 10u.

6.1.3.2. Gill Flagellates

In recent years fish of different species, especially cichlids, have been repeatedly examined to study the massive infestation of their gills with flagellates of the genus *Cryptobia*, presumably *Cryptobia branchialis*. In severe infections of the gills, the pathogens also can be found in skin smears from the flanks of the fish. They cannot be distinguished from the *Cryptobia* that occur in the intestines. They have possibly developed from *Cryptobia branchialis* (see Chapter 6.1.2). Treatment is according to method C_8 or C_{1c}.

6.1.3.3. *Oodinium*

Oodinium pillularis, the cause of velvet disease, is a dinoflagellate that in its parasitic phase on the fish can attain a size of more than 100 microns, making it just visible as a light spot with the naked eye. The skin, gills,

and often intestines are affected. Seen from the front longitudinally against the light, the surface appears dull. In severe infections the fish takes on a velvety texture, the coating looking yellow to yellowish brown. The skin may come off in pieces (Photograph No. 9, Chart 5). Inflammations and fungal overgrowths rarely occur. Severe infection of the gills causes the fish to breathe hard, even though the rest of the skin may be free of parasites. Microscopic examination under at least 100X reveals roundish to elongated cells of a yellowish brown color resting with their narrow end on the mucosa. Clusters of large and small cells often occur like grapes (Photograph No. 75). An elliptical cell nucleus apparently made of many small bodies often can be recognized against the brownish protoplasma. The rootlet-like protoplasmal filaments (rhizoids) that anchor in the skin of the fish are difficult to recognize unless stained (Photograph No. 76). With these the parasite destroys the skin cells of the fish, taking their content as food. This sessile parasitic phase of *Oodinium* lacks flagella, thus depriving the parasite of any resemblance to flagellates.

When the *Oodinium* cell has taken enough nutrient it drops off, falling to the bottom of the aquarium, where it contracts and begins to di-

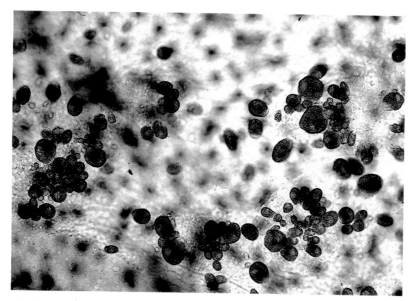

75. *Oodinium pillularis* in groups on the skin.

vide. The daughter cells formed in this way divide several times shortly afterward, forming 30 to 200 flagellated cells. They are almost round and have a longitudinal as well as a transverse groove, at the intersection of which originate two flagella. Only one projects from the surface of the cell and provides locomotion. A red eyespot is easier to discern than the longitudinal groove. The average diameter is 15 microns, with a 30% variation.

These flagellated "dinospores" can live free for only 24 hours at most, dying if they do not find a host within this time. Once they do find a host fish, they attach themselves to it and drop the flagella. The parasite harms the fish with its root-like filaments, the rhizoids, which penetrate into the epithelial cells and loosen fragments for nutrients. The cellular integrity of the skin is destroyed and the tissue dies. Even hemorrhages can occur in the gill filaments. An *Oodinium* infection runs for many weeks until the skin is massively covered with the parasites and disintegrates, slowly killing the fish. Treatment is according to method B_1, C_4, or C_{13}.

Oodinium limneticum is similar to *Oodinium pillularis*, but there is no red eyespot in the dinospores. It has been found only in North America.

Oodinoides vastator forms a large, bright, blister-like parasitic phase that occurs on inflamed skin in tropical fish. Its dinospores are green. The coral fish disease, *Oodinium ocellatum,* has been known for 50 years. It occurs in marine aquariums, where newly imported fish are often affected. Its appearance and development are similar to those of *Oodinium pil-*

76. *Oodinium pillularis.* Isolated specimens. Size: 74u.

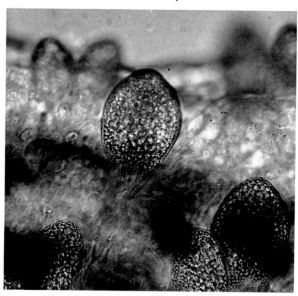

lularis. The parasitic phases contain starch granules that can be identified by the addition of iodine. Treatment is according to method B_1, C_4, or C_{13}. When treatment of seawater is with copper sulfate, it must usually be repeated on the third or fourth day. Observe the fish so as to be able to take countermeasures in case of an overdose. Also refer to the instructions in Chapter 10, method C_{13}.

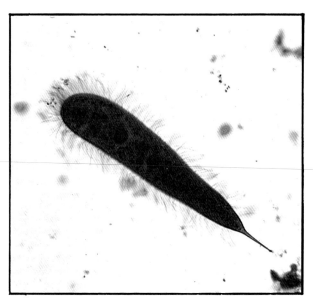

77. *Protoopalina symphysodonis.* Size: 118u. Carbol fuchsin stain.

6.1.4. Opalinids, Discus Parasite *Protoopalina*

Opalinids are real giants among the flagellates. Because of their average size of 0.1 mm and the innumerable flagella distributed over all of the cell surface, they are easily confused with ciliates. They were first discovered in the gut of amphibians, then later in the intestine of fish from the upper Nile, and in discus *(Symphysodon).* Opalinids in fish have not yet been definitely shown to be real parasites.

It has been more than ten years now since Dr. Schubert reported ciliate-like protozoa in the gut of discus. The scientific name of the giant parasites that were at first called "discus parasites" is *Protoopalina symphysodonis.* They often attain a length of 0.12 mm, with a ratio of length to width of between 6:1.5 and

6:0.9. The difference is due to the organisms being thinner following division. The discus parasites reproduce vegetatively by longitudinal division. There probably is sexual reproduction, but it has not yet been demonstrated. The anterior pole is round and often angled to the major axis of the body. The posterior pole forms a spine-like point. The flagella are arranged in rows that spiral around the cell. The cell protoplasm contains many tiny vacuoles and two equally large nuclei, one behind the other (Photograph No. 77). The movements of discus parasites are rapid and gliding, turning around the long axis. Sudden stops and backward swimming are just as possible. Since ingestion of nutrients occurs over the whole cell surface, there is no gullet.

A moderate infection causes only minimal damage to discus. A more precise prognosis on the effect of the parasite is impossible because a mixed infection with *Spironucleus* or parasitic worms is generally present. Only on one occasion was it observed that a discus population perished from a severe infection of only *Protoopalina symphysodonis (Zool. Anz., Jena,* 202, 1979). Large discus, even when heavily infested, usually do not show any signs or symptoms of disease. Smaller juveniles may have their growth stunted. Transmission to other fish is only slight, since parasites in water suitable for breeding discus die of plasmolysis in two hours at the most. Transmission is possible only if the freshly dropped feces of an infected fish are ingested. Diagnosis is made by microscopic (200X) examination of very fresh feces. Treatment with Metronidazol according to method C_{19} definitely kills discus parasites.

6.2. Amoebae

In recent years parasitic amoebae have been found in marine fish, trout, salmon, and other fish of cold waters. Gills, intestines, and other organs were affected, many fish dying of the infections. To what extent amoebae can be dangerous to warm-water fish is still not known. An emaciated discus slightly affected with flagellates was found to contain a large quantity of amoebae in its gut, but this was an isolated case. Treatment according to C_8 can be successful.

6.3. Sporozoa

Sporozoan infections do not occur very often in aquariums. A disease caused by one of these protozoans is often known as "neon tetra disease"; the pathogen is *Pleistophora hyphessobryconis.* All sporozoans are parasites, occurring in the internal organs as well as on the skin and in muscle tissue. Adaptation to a parasitic life has deprived most of the species of their motility. Sporozoans infect freshwater as well as marine fish.

Many sporozoan species cause small nodules in the skin, gills, or internal organs, ranging in size from a few microns to 2 millimeters. The spores are released by squashing the nodules on a microscope slide. Inside the spores, seen at very high power, are up to four strongly refractive bodies, the polar capsules. Nodules in skin and fins can be confused with

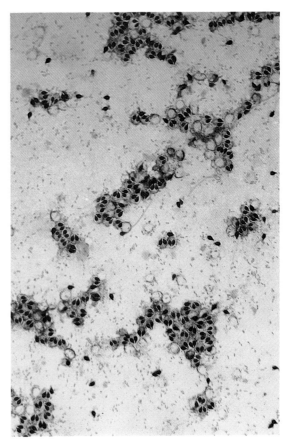

79. Spores of a *Myxosporan* stained with E_9. Length: 12u.

78. *Eimeria* spp. spore capsules from chocolate gourami *(Sphaerichthys osphromenoides).* Size: 12-14u.

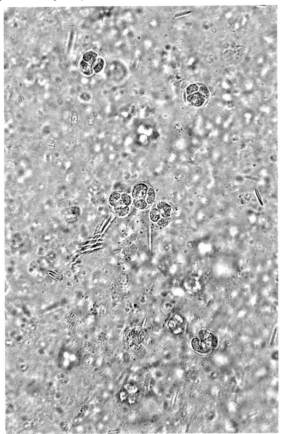

lymphocystis (Chapter 4.1). To confirm the diagnosis, sporozoan spores (which do not occur in lymphocystis) must be found. Sporozoan infections can affect all exotic or ornamental fish but do not occur very often. The pathogens are often introduced into the aquarium along with fish captured in the wild. Cold-water fish caught in streams and ponds also can be affected. The following sections deal briefly with several sporozoan diseases that can be introduced along with cold-water fish.

6.3.1. Coccidia

Coccidian diseases normally occur only in carp but were found in sticklebacks by G. Schmidt. Various genera occur in the gut, air bladder, liver, and blood. *Eimeria* spp. form spore-containing cysts (oocysts) up to 40 microns in size (Photograph No. 78). The ones that parasitize blood attack the blood corpuscles and, once inside them, can be seen as elongated structures beside the cell nucleus. Treatment according to method C_{22} can be tried.

6.3.2. Myxospora

Myxospora are widely distributed in cold-water fish, causing whirling disease. The fish are affected by disequilibrium. Cysts are found in many organs and contain myxosporidia spores averaging 10 microns in size. They are visible at both spindle-shaped polar capsules (Photograph No. 79). The disease runs a very slow course, taking months. As it continues it causes deformation, nodules, boils, and a dark coloration of the posterior third of the fish. Prepare mounts of skin, gills, and internal organs and examine them for nodules, which can range in size from 50 to several hundred microns. Large numbers of spores are released—and are visible at the polar capsules—when the cysts are squashed. Since no treatment is known, affected fish are sacrificed and the aquarium disinfected.

80. Spores of a *Microspora* genus, probably *Glugea,* from an African climbing perch ("bush" fish). Size: 5u.

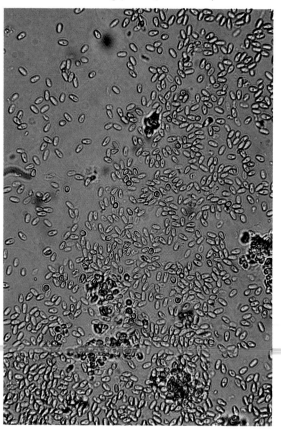

6.3.3. Microspora

Various genera of microsporidians cause disease in cold-water fish. The species *Glugea anomala,* for example, occurs in sticklebacks, forming white 10-mm cysts in intestines, testes, air bladder wall, and connective tissue. Boils formed just under the skin appear to be attached. The parasites are in these cysts. The spores are oval, often egg-shaped, measuring 3 x 2 microns (Photograph No. 80). No method of treatment is known.

6.3.3.1. *Pleistophora*

Pleistophora (also spelled *Plistophora)* also is a microsporidian genus. These pathogens parasitize the muscle strands, forming spherical cysts (pansporoblasts) gathered closely together within small areas. They occur in marine and freshwater fish. In the aquarium, *Pleistophora hyphessobryconis* occurs as the cause of neon tetra disease. Besides neons *(Paracheirodon innesi),* other characid species and various cold-water fish are affected, except for the cardinal tetra *(Paracheirodon axelrodi).*

The disease is manifested by pale coloration and white areas. In the neon, the color band is broken. The fish swim restlessly around at night, sometimes also exhibiting vertebral deformations as secondary symptoms. Teased specimens of affected muscle reveal masses of pansporoblasts, easily recognized by their dark coloration (Photograph No. 32, Chart 18). The 30-micron pansporoblasts contain many 4-micron to 7-micron spores that are liberated after the cysts rupture (Photograph No. 81). In the aquarium, the spores are ingested as the fish feed. The amoebid embryo hatches in the intestine, penetrates through the intestinal wall, and forms new pansporoblasts in the musculature. The affected muscle strands become necrotic and turn white. If diseased and dead fish are not removed from the aquarium, an outbreak of epidemic proportions is possible. No reliable treatment is known.

6.4. Ciliates

Compared with the parasites described up to now, the ciliates are very large protozoa. Many species are provided with a thick covering of

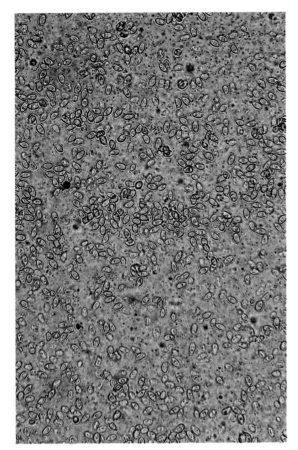

81. *Plistophora* spores from *Macropodus chinensis*. Size: 7u.

coordinately motile cilia over the whole body surface, thus giving this group of organisms its name. The most important characteristic, however, is the presence of two nuclei. The macronucleus controls cell function and the micronucleus controls sexual functions. Although the firm cellular membrane lends a characteristic shape to the cell, it can be radically modified for short periods.

6.4.1. *Ichthyophthirius multifiliis*

"White spot disease," "sand grain or gravel disease," or simply "ich" is what many aquarium hobbyists call this disease. When heavily infected, the fish is covered with so many white spots that it looks as if it were sprinkled with grit, gravel, or coarse sand, (Photograph No. 7, Chart 5). The fish rapidly rub up against solid objects as they swim horizontally, attempting to free themselves of the parasites. Eventually they become lethargic and apa-

thetic. Then white spots appear and large pieces of the skin begin to disintegrate, representing the terminal stage just preceding death. The parasites hold on, constantly turning between the epidermis and the dermis, nourishing themselves from the components of the destroyed skin cells and the body fluid. The parasites stimulate the skin lying above them to proliferate, forming a protective covering.

The size of *I. multifiliis* ranges between 0.5 and 1.5 millimeters. In a smear mount the parasite usually is spherical. The cell surface is covered with several thousand small cilia that produce a constant twisting movement. Ich cells are good swimmers in open water. The large horseshoe-shaped nucleus can be easily recognized if food particles do not cloud the protoplasm (Photograph No. 82).

The grown parasite lets go of its host and actively swims around looking for a quiet area of water where it can reproduce. It attaches itself to an object and then encloses itself in a viscous capsule, within which it divides into two cells, then four, etc., until up to a thousand swarmer cells are formed within eight to 24 hours. The time depends upon the water temperature (Photograph No. 83). The swarmer cells, 30 to 50 microns in size, are good swimmers because of their cilia. They leave the

82. Isolated specimen of *Ichthyophthirius multifiliis*. Bright field photograph. Size 552u.

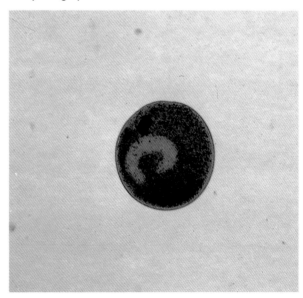

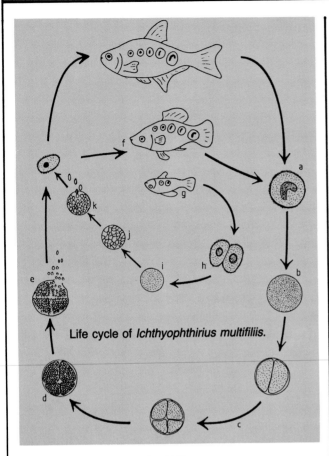

Life cycle of *Ichthyophthirius multifiliis.*

83. THE VICIOUS ICH CYCLE

Ich is probably the most widespread and common of all fish diseases, It is variously referred to as Ich, White Spot or Salt-and-pepper Disease. It is caused by the parasite *Ichthyophthirius multifiliis.*

A. The white spot cyst on the fish has matured and left the host. B. The cell begins to ripen. C. First it divides into two parts. It continues dividing by cell division process to 4, then 8, then 16, etc. D. After about 20 hours the mother cell is full and will soon rupture, releasing the daughter cells. E. The mother cell ruptures. F. The daughter cells, which are free-swimming, have 48 hours to find a fish host or they perish. G. They leave fish which have died. H. Two to three days later mature parasites mate (conjugation) for sexual reproduction. I. They produce cysts which can live for several weeks in the aquarium without finding a host. J. Eventually the cysts hatch and start the mother-daughter cell cycle once again. K. The new parasites start searching for a suitable host and the cycle is complete.

cysts and actively swim in search of a new host fish. If none is found within 48 hours, they die. Cell division of the swarmer cells is still possible even after they leave the cysts (Photograph No. 84). At first round to oval in shape, they assume an elongated to oval shape with age.

Once a swarmer cell finds a host fish, it penetrates the skin and stays between the epidermis and dermis, where it grows for ten to 20 days and builds up its substance for the next division. The time the parasite needs to grow larger in the skin depends upon two factors: the water temperature and the fish's resistance.

Ichthyophthirius organisms attacking for the first time have a longer growth phase than those that affect an already severely infected fish. If the affected fish dies, all the parasites abandon the skin over the course of the next few hours. Regardless of what size they may have attained, they form a cystic capsule and begin to divide. The smallest specimens go through a sexual process (conjugation) to form a permanent or resting stage that is viable for several weeks.

After surviving an infection, the fish are, to a certain extent, immune to further infection. The parasites then form a latent stage at protected sites such as gills or fin bases. Subsequent stress, poor conditions, or transfer causes these stages to reactivate and attack the same or even newly introduced fish. Newly purchased fish thus can suddenly become infected, and the aquarium keeper will erroneously believe that he has introduced parasites with the new fish. The truth is, however, that the new fish—not yet immune to the parasite—were infected by the latent stages of the parasite already waiting in the tank. In such a case the seller is often unfairly blamed.

Treatment of an already started infection can consist of raising the temperature to 28°-30°C if the fish can tolerate that increase. This heat treatment must last at least three weeks (method B_1). The transfer method (B_2) is time-consuming and weakens the fish. Chemical treatment can be with compounds containing malachite green. Methods C_1, C_4, and C_{16} also are effective.

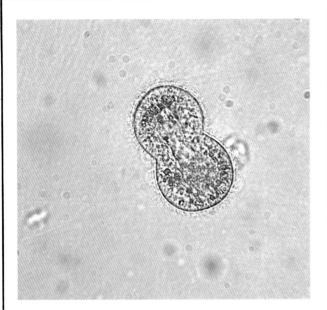

84. The swarm spores often go on dividing even after leaving the cyst.

6.4.2. Cryptocaryon irritans

The symptoms of "marine ich" can easily be confused with those of *Ichthyophthirius.* The fish is covered with pale spots ranging in shade from white to gray that are not easy to simply brush off. In the beginning stage the fish rubs itself, its coloration fades, and the skin clouds over. The course of the disease drags on. The white nodules represent epithelial growths in which the parasite lives. In severe infections they can be grouped together or they can coalesce over the surface. The course is then marked by tissue destruction, hemorrhages, inflammations, and skin disintegration. Bacterial and fungal infections can add to the problem.

Cryptocaryon attacks all species of marine fish. The fish are blinded when the parasites attach to the eyes. If not treated on time, the fish succumb within five days of the appearance of the spots.

The parasite measures from 0.5 to 2 mm. It is round to pear-shaped. The cell membrane is fully ciliated. The macronucleus consists of four round parts usually arranged in an arc. To obtain living specimens for a mount requires very careful work, since the firmly attached parasite in the skin of the host fish can easily be destroyed by the pressure needed to remove it. Just like *Ichthyophthirius, Cryptocaryon* drops off the host after the growth phase, falls to the bottom, and forms a capsule around itself. After six to nine days, more than 200 35-micron swarmer cells leave the cyst. They have only 24 hours to find a host, otherwise they die. Treatment is according to method C_{14} or C_{15}.

6.4.3. Chilodonella cyprini

This large heart-shaped organism parasitizes skin and gills. The fish rub themselves against objects and become lethargic. When the gills are involved, they hang just under the surface and gasp for air. The area from back of the head to the dorsal fins seems to be a preferred site. First, 0.5 to 1 mm round or elliptical spots on the skin become cloudy. The skin thickens at these well-defined areas and the color fades to white. Finally it begins to disintegrate. Small, young, and weak fish can become affected uniformly over the whole body, in which case they die. The gills sometimes are destroyed as far back as the solid cartilage. In stronger, more resistant fish, only white, slimy areas form on the skin and enlarge only very little over the course of several days (Photograph No. 8, Chart 5).

In the microscopic preparation of the skin smear, ciliates can be seen that measure 50 microns on the average and have a notch on the posterior pole, giving them a heart-shaped appearance. Only the upper side is uniformly ciliated, the underside having just a few rows of cilia (Photograph No. 85). The parasite can swim and thus can reach other fish. A thickly populated tank favors the spread of the disease. The parasites reproduce by division into two. Introduction into the aquarium can occur along with live food from fish ponds. Prevention consists of clean food and not too many fish in the tank. In mild cases, methods C_{12} and C_{1a} suffice; greater effect is provided by methods C_{1c}, C_{17a}, and C_{16}.

6.4.4. Brooklynella hostilis

Brooklynella hostilis has been recognized during the last few years as a parasite of tropical marine fish. The fish most at risk are those under stress and those living in overpopulated aquariums and polluted water. Under these

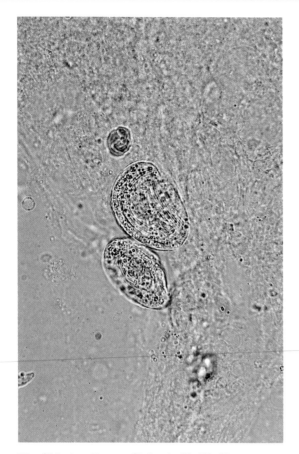

85. *Chilodonella* spp. Stained with E6. Size: 50u.

conditions the disease can assume epidemic proportions. The pathogen, *Brooklynella hostilis,* is a holotrichous (completely ciliated) ciliate of the family Dysteriidae. It looks and develops very much like the freshwater parasite *Chilodonella. Brooklynella* lives on the skin and gills of fish, nourishing itself from skin and blood cells. The infection begins with small pale areas that grow larger until the epithelium comes off in sheets. The fish loses its appetite, swims slowly, secretes mucus, and breathes heavily. Death occurs in several days if large skin areas are destroyed.

Skin and gill smears, as well as smears from lesions, are taken for diagnosis. This heart-shaped parasite attains an average size of 60 microns. On the abdominal or ventral side is a holding organ for attachment to the fish. Just as in many other ciliates, *Brooklynella* is heavily ciliated and can swim rapidly as well as maneuverably. The parasite is in most cases in-

troduced into the aquarium along with infected fish. It quickly reproduces under the conditions described above. For prevention, we can only recommend—just as we do in the case of all parasites that attack weak hosts—keeping the aquarium hygienic and not exposing the fish to any stress. G. Blasiola recommends briefly dipping newly acquired and suspect fish into freshwater; the pH must be exactly that of the seawater. Depending upon species, the bath should not last longer than one to five minutes. Treatment with copper is useless. Methods C_{16} b and C_7 are other treatment possibilities.

6.4.5. *Trichodina*

When the fish rub and scrape themselves or jerk violently with their fins, they could be affected with *Trichodina* spp. There is usually nothing on the skin to see. A few parasites do not hurt the fish, but a heavy infestation leads to the formation of whitish spots on the skin. *Trichodina* no doubt occurs in an aquarium

86. *Trichodina* spp. Stained with E10. Size 50u.

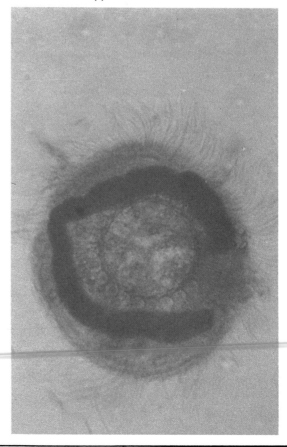

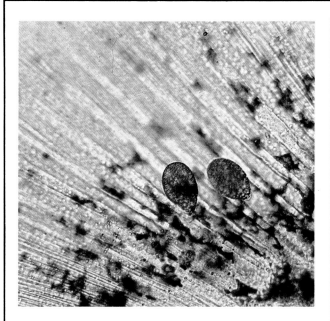

87. *Tetrahymena pyriformis* on the tail fin of a young fish. Size 80u.

more often than previously believed, because their sporadic presence usually is not noted. When the organism is suspected, take smears from several places and examine at 100 to 200X.

The pathogen is a highhat-shaped ciliate crowned with a ring of cilia at each pole of the cylindrical cell. A ring of hooks is on the underside. When the parasite lies flat in the mount, the rings of hooks and cilia are sharply delineated (Photograph No. 86). *Trichodina* spins constantly and can quickly change from place to place on the fish. The average diameter of the cell is 50 microns.

Recent studies (Hausmann, 1981) have demonstrated that *Trichodina* is not a real parasite. This ciliate uses the fish merely for transportation, holding on to the skin with a holding disc and a ring of hooks. It feeds on bacteria. The gullet is on the side opposite the fish. Because increased numbers of bacteria show up when the skin is injured, the *Trichodina,* too, can multiply well. Their sucking discs damage the skin even more. Even in clean aquariums large numbers of bacteria are available to *Trichodina,* which can then multiply well. They do this by division. *Trichodina* swims freely from fish to fish. Here, too, the source of infection is often food from ponds.

Control is effected by method C_{17a}, C_{16}, or C_{1b}, according to the severity of the infection.

6.4.6. Other Ciliates

Ciliates that are really not parasites are often found on fish in heavily contaminated water. Since aquarium water is usually more contaminated than the native waters of the fish, these ciliates belong to the normal population of the aquarium. They can increase prodigiously in neglected tanks. Numbers of them can be found on weakened fish. Fungus-covered wounds and skin sites damaged by other parasites are preferred feeding grounds for them because of all the bacteria there. Countermeasures include hygienic measures and removal of wounded fish to a quarantine tnak.

Tetrahymena pyriformis is one of these ciliates (Photograph No. 87). It is pear-shaped (pyriform), 35 to 90 microns in size, and appears in large numbers at infected skin sites. Affected fish fold up their fins and rock their

88. *Paramecium.* Size: 100-150u. Many ciliates live in aquarium water and feed predominantly on bacteria.

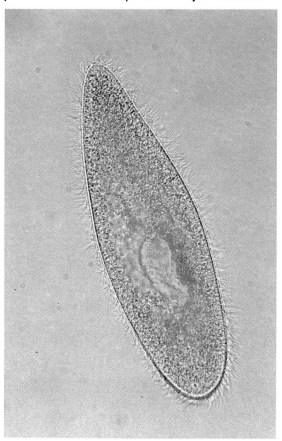

bodies. After control of the primary disease, *Tetrahymena* can be controlled with method C_{16}.

Great numbers of *Vorticella* (Photograph No. 89) often sit with their retractable stalk on damaged skin, which they can damage even more by attacking their stalk. Paramecia (Photograph No. 88) search for their main diet of bacteria in the filter, in the bottom debris, and in decomposing fecal matter.

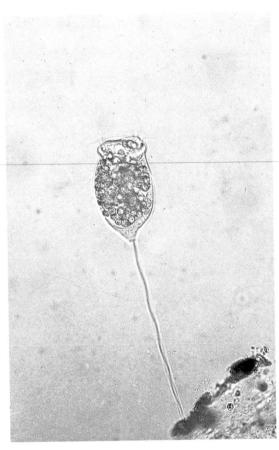

89. *Vorticella* form a long stem which can suddenly contract. Size: 50-150u.

Chapter 7
WORM DISEASES

There are so many species of parasitic worms that an all-encompassing description is impossible in this context. We will deal mainly with species that are common and can threaten aquarium fish. Worm diseases generally take a slow course and often are accompanied by other diseases, so the cause of death usually cannot be ascribed with complete certainty to worms.

7.1. Turbellaria

Planarians, common free-living flatworms, are rare as fish parasites, and only few cases have been reported up to now of planarians parasitizing the skin of marine fish or lower animals. They often, however, appear as egg thieves in aquariums. They can multiply well when the bottom is full of debris. When it gets dark, they attack the eggs. They can be controlled by vacuuming out the debris during the weekly change of water. According to Reichenbach-Klinke, they can be controlled by adding two tablespoons of vinegar to 25 liters of water.

7.2. Monogenetic Trematodes or Flukes

7.2.1. Hookworms

Hookworms live on the skin and gills of freshwater and marine fish. The grasping hooks on the posterior end serve to hold on to the skin of the host. A general identification can be made from the number and shape of grasping hooks, and that is often necessary for an aquarium hobbyist because control of the various species is not always attainable with the same methods. Fish tolerate a mild infestation well, though sometimes they rub or scrape themselves and jerk their fins. In heavy infestations, the opercula are spread out. Slime formation on the gills hinders breathing, causing rapid breathing (Photograph No. 23, Chart 10). The fish hang just under the surface of the water and breathe heavily. Sometimes one operculum is open, the other laid back, and the mouth puckered. In extreme cases the oxygen uptake is so reduced that the fish die.

Hookworms are usually host-specific, so that only closely related fish species are affected. In heavily populated breeding tanks, gill worms can multiply to epidemic proportions, killing off the whole population of young fish within a few weeks. In suspected cases, prepare skin and gill smears, which will show the worms well at 50 to 200X. They attach

90. *Gyrodactylus* spp. with embryo. Moderate size (0.6mm).

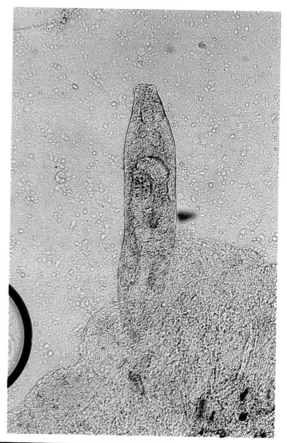

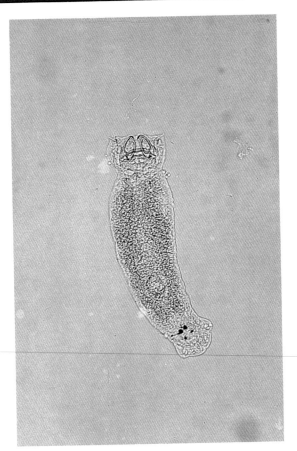

91. Gill worm of the Dactilogyridea family with four central hooks. Size: 0.3mm

provided with hooks usually is visible inside the middle section of the worm. This embryo itself contains a young embryo with still another embryo, thus four generations are joined in one parent. Although *Gyrodactylus* species give birth to only one worm at one time, the reproduction rate is very high. A sexually mature worm could, under favorable conditions, produce about one million young within one month (Schäperclaus, 1979).

The worms nourish themselves by scraping and sucking for blood and skin fragments. A few individuals will not damage the fish. Only when unfavorable conditions weaken the fish does a massive multiplication of the parasite become possible. Large skin lesions with cloudiness result, opening the way for bacterial and fungal infections. *Gyrodactylus* species, because of their host-specificity, do not represent any danger to fish in well-managed aquariums. If, however, massive reproduction does occur, look for the reason for the weakness in the fish (another disease, stress, etc.; see Chapter 2). Worms that drop off can live for five to ten days without any fish host. In practice, it is not necessary to differentiate among the various *Gyrodactylus* species. It is important, however, to recognize them as such. Treatment is simple and can be according to methods C_{18}, C_{11}, and C_7. Since there are no eggs, a one-time treatment suffices.

strongly to the fish skin by their grasping hooks and move their anterior ends to and fro. Whole gill arches can be removed from fish that have just died and examined at 50X to reveal large numbers of worms. Hookworms are introduced along with new fish that are added to the aquarium and also are transmitted by parents even to their smallest fry.

7.2.1.1. Gyrodactylidea

Gyrodactylus spp. parasitize the skin and more rarely the gills. Transmission to other fish is favored by overpopulation. Microscopically, 50 to 200X immediately reveals the hook organs on the posterior end of the 0.3 to 0.9 mm worms (Photograph No. 90). The posterior disc contains two central hooks surrounded by 16 smaller hooks. The anterior end is forked and contains the outlet of the glue glands. A sucker is located posteriorly and ventrally. There are no eyespots. An embryo already

7.2.1.2. Dactylogyridea

Monogenetic flukes or trematodes of the order Dactylogyridea live mainly on gills. They measure between 0.1 and 2 mm and possess a doubly forked anterior end with a sucker and four or more black eyespots. The holding organ at the posterior end contains, depending on the species, two or four central hooks, plus 12, 14, or 16 peripheral hooks (Photograph No. 91). Their lifespan ranges from 12 days to several months. Without a host, they can survive only two to eight days.

Diagnosis requires noting whether, in the four-hook worms, the hooks are connected by one or two strips or bands. If two are present, then we are dealing with gill worms of a still not completely known genus that mainly parasitizes discus fish (Photograph No. 92). To

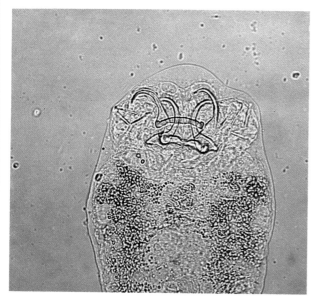

92. Gill worm of the Dactilogyridea family. Holding organ with four central hooks.

show the hook organ well, mounts have to be thin so the worms lie still (Chapter 11.4 to 11.6). To gather enough worms for mounting, remove the gill arches and place them in a small dish filled with aquarium water. In one to two hours, lift the arches out with forceps and pipette up all the worms that dropped off the gills and fell to the bottom of the dish.

The Dactylogyridea are hermaphroditic. After mutual fertilization, a relatively large egg forms in each worm. A smear reveals an oval egg with a small thorn-like projection on the shell. An egg measures about 50 microns (Photograph No. 93). Most of the eggs become detached from the gills, but a few hang on. Development takes a few hours to four days, then a ciliated larva emerges and actively swims off in search of a fish host.

The four eyespots allow the larva to discern light and shadow. It perceives the fish as shadow, swims to it, and attaches itself to the body of the fish. Over the next two days it climbs slowly forward over the skin toward the gills. When it reaches the gills it takes three to six days until it attains sexual maturity. Because of this behavior it is not necessary to take a smear directly from the gills. A smear from about 0.5 to 1 cm behind the operculum on the side of the body is sufficient.

In the smear, larvae can be seen microscopically at 200 and 400X. In another four to five days the larvae develop into adult worms with a life expectancy of still another eight days. Larvae can survive one day without a fish host, the adults up to six days. Many *Dactylogyrus* eggs are sensitive to dryness. As dangerous as a *Dactylogyrus* infection can be to young fish, it is harmless to vigorous, healthy adult fish. The fish evidently develops resistance to gill worms when half-grown. Since, however, a certain number of worms remain latent on the gills, they can multiply if the host fish weakens and loses resistance, which then also threatens its tankmates.

If you find gill worms in a school of discus that you bred yourself, then it can be assumed they were infected from the parent fish. Even later broods will infect themselves during the time they feed on the parents' skin mucus. Gill worms multiply so rapidly that they can destroy a whole brood within six weeks. That has become a problem in discus breeding. The Dactylogyridea of discus are 0.2 to 0.3 mm long (Photograph No. 91). Their four central hooks measure 33 microns (Photograph No. 92). Since the worms can also survive on other species of fish, transmission is possible via newly introduced fish in the aquarium.

93. *Dactylogyrus* spp. egg with thornlike outgrowth. Size 40u.

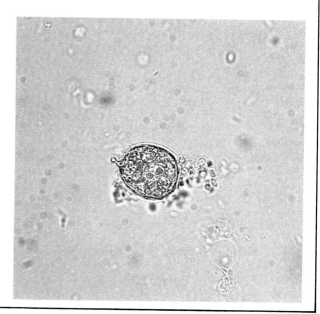

They have already been found on characins, catfish, and even on livebearers. Even if these other species were kept some time ago with the discus, even for a short period, worms were still found. The worms are not resistant to Masoten (methiphonate, trichlorphone), as is often assumed; only their eggs are resistant. Since some of these remain on the bottom and develop later, even three applications of treatment according to method C_{18a} do not give more than briefly successful results. The eggs perish quickly under dry conditions, so they can be eliminated by drying out the tank for three days. Treatment according to C_{18c} frees one aquarium population of the parasite. Treatment with method C_6 is more reliable. The fish should be observed regularly to catch any developing problems.

When discus parents are known to harbor gill worms, the young must receive preventive treatment after the parents are removed. Even if the breeding couple do not show any signs of infestation, many gill worms may be living on them. Treatment according to methods C_7 and C_{11} are effective only when the treated fish are not returned to the aquarium. An aquarium free of gill worms can be obtained by regular application of method C_{18c} or C_6.

7.2.2. Other Skin and Gill Worms

There is another whole series of gill and skin worms of various forms and sizes that infest freshwater and marine fish. They are usually introduced with live foods or specimens captured in the wild but do not multiply very much in the aquarium because they are specialized for one species of fish. Many of these worms lay eggs that anchor to the gills by means of a filament. Since usually only a few eggs are laid, there is no danger of any serious multiplication. Sometimes diplozoons or twin-worms appear on the gills of freshwater fish. They can be recognized by their characteristic "Siamese-twin" form, two individuals having grown together at midbody for life. Their reproductive rate is extremely slow because they lay only one egg at a time. Gill irritation can occur. Treatment is according to method C_{18}, C_{11}, or C_7.

7.3. Digenetic Trematodes or Flukes

Digenetic flatworms are parasites of the internal organs of freshwater and marine fish. They need one or two intermediate hosts to complete their life cycles. The fish can be the definitive or the intermediate host. If the fish is an end host, the parasites are mainly in the intestine or stomach. Their powerful suction discs can damage the intestinal wall. Many digenetic trematodes can grow large enough to obstruct the intestines in smaller fish hosts. Further damage is inflicted when the worms feed. The worms deposit their eggs in the intestines, from where they are eliminated with the feces into open water. Then the ciliated larvae (the miracida) hatch and begin searching for their first intermediate host, usually a snail or other invertebrate. After growth they leave the intermediate host and are now cercariae, recognizable by their forked tail. The fish ingest the cercariae along with the food. In the fish's intestines they cast off their tail and develop into the parasitic worm stage or encapsulate as metacercariae (Photograph No. 94). In the latter case the fish is the second intermediate host and fish-eating birds or mammals become the definitive hosts.

Other trematodes go through an asexual division, forming sporocysts, some of which then form rediae, which finally produce great numbers of cercariae that abandon their snail hosts and seek out a fish host. On the fish host they penetrate the skin and spread to all possible organs (Photograph No. 33, Chart 20). Many encapsulate right under the scales, appearing as large (0.5 to 1 mm) black dots (black spot disease). Encapsulated metacercariae cause blindness when they occur in the fish's eye.

In the aquarium, digenetic trematode infestations are rare. Fish captured in the wild often bring encapsulated metacercariae along with them. Introduction of the disease is only by means of snails, therefore they should not be brought in from open-air ponds. Since water birds feed from even the smallest bodies of water, snails from fish-free ponds also represent a danger. If you insist on having snails, let some deposit their eggs in a glass jar, then transfer those to the aquarium. Infected fish cannot be cured.

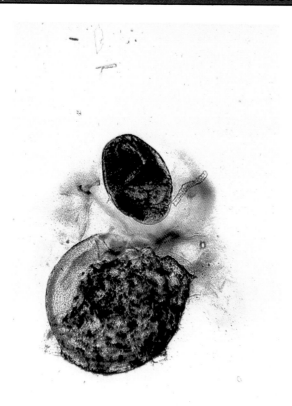

94. Open metacercarial cyst with worm larva cyst. Size: 740u.

7.4. Cestodes or Tapeworms

The tapeworms also reach sexual maturity by passing through intermediate hosts. The first stage occurs in copepods or tubificid worms. The fish can be either an intermediate or a definitive host. Their life cycle is similar to that of Digenea, therefore there is no need to go into it again. Tapeworms occur in freshwater and marine fish (Photograph No. 95) but are rare in aquariums. Their occurrence is limited to specimens captured in the wild, in which worms and larvae (procercoids) can be found. They may show up in the intestine as worm-like larvae or in any organs as encapsulated cysts. Despite the danger that tapeworm larvae could be introduced along with tubifex worms and cyclops, which I have regularly fed to my fish for years, I have never found any cestodes in my tanks. Larva cannot be detected in the living fish, but the presence of sexually mature adults can be recognized by their eggs and detached segments, which appear in the fish feces (Photograph No. 96). Treatment is possible only with oral medication according to method C_{24}, which has to be repeated until the head (scolex) of the tapeworm is eliminated with the feces.

Trematodes of the genus *Sanguinicola* (bloodworms) live in the fish's circulatory system. Their eggs are carried by the bloodstream into the gill capillaries, where they stick tight, often blocking the capillary. The emerging larva (miracidium) penetrates through the gill tissue to gain access to open water, where it then seeks an intermediate host (snails of the family Lymnaeidae). The cercariae, which abandon the snail after a while, penetrate into a fish and develop to sexual maturity within the vascular system. Bloodworms and their eggs are demonstrable in the gills. Encapsulated eggs can be found in the kidneys. Affected fish are lethargic and have pale gills. Treatment can be attempted with method C_{24}, but success is uncertain. If there are no snails in the aquarium, the parasite cannot spread.

95. Tapeworm from the gut of a *discus* fish. Length: 5cm.

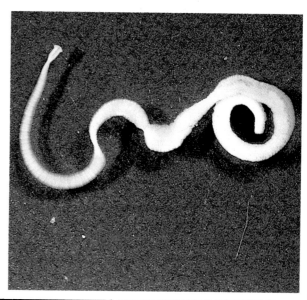

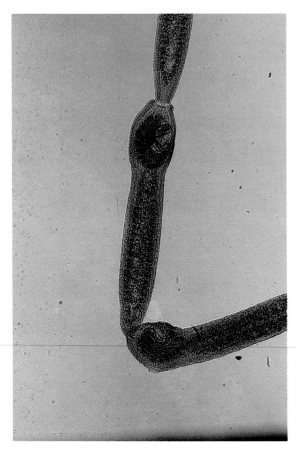

96. Tapeworm segments found in the droppings of a ray, *Potamotrygon laticeps*. Mounted and stained with E4. Length of each segment 2.8-3mm.

7.5. Nematodes or Roundworms

Roundworms are frequent parasites of freshwater fish in the aquarium. In marine tanks they may be introduced along with new fish, but they cannot reproduce because their development requires an intermediate host. At autopsy the larvae are found encapsulated in the tissues. Newly captured freshwater fish also can sometimes harbor nematode cysts (Photograph No. 34, Chart 20). There is danger only if both the intermediate and the definitive hosts are kept in the same aquarium. Various organs can be infected with the nematodes of their larvae. Isolated parasites inconvenience the host very little. Heavy infestation emaciates the host, producing a "knifeback" or "razorback" condition showing a sharp ridge under the emaciated dorsal skin. The fish dies when an organ ceases to function.

As a rule, other infections (various pathogens such as flagellates and bacteria) join in, so the cause of death is often uncertain.

Tropical freshwater nematodes without alternating hosts stand a good chance of spreading in an aquarium. The unsegmented body has a round, spindle-shaped, or thread-like cross-section. Great length in a nematode may be associated with thinness *(Capillaria).*

7.5.1. *Capillaria* (Filarial worms)

Capillaria is an intestinal parasite of freshwater fish (Photograph No. 97), which can tolerate a mild infestation. When the worms have multiplied heavily, however, the fish begin to stand off alone, become emaciated, and sometimes stop eating. Diagnosis can be made from a fecal smear, in which *Capillaria* eggs can be seen at 300 to 400X (Photograph No. 20, Chart 8). They differ from species to species but often resemble a cylinder with rounded ends or are oval. The ends look like they are stoppered, which is characteristic; the "stoppers" may look like champagne corks or only small protuberances. A very mild infection is defined by finding not more than three to five eggs in each of several centimeter-long fecal strands. The worms themselves can only be found by dissecting the fresh intestine. They move constantly; immobile specimens are dead. These nematodes are often longer than a centimeter, but they are thinner than a human hair (that is why the German word for them means "hairworm"). To examine them better, dissect out the intestines, cut them open longitudinally under water (physiological saline), and with a dissecting needle transfer the worms to a microscope slide. Inside the female the consecutively aligned eggs can be recognized at 150X (Photograph No. 97). The eggs gain access to the water by dropping out with the feces and lying on the bottom, where they develop partially. Only when they are ingested by a fish do they complete their development and hatch in the intestine. The disease spreads very slowly. Outbreaks of epidemic proportions and losses occur only rarely. The fish, in that case, are most certainly also infected with other diseases as well. *Capillaria* is rarely introduced with live foods.

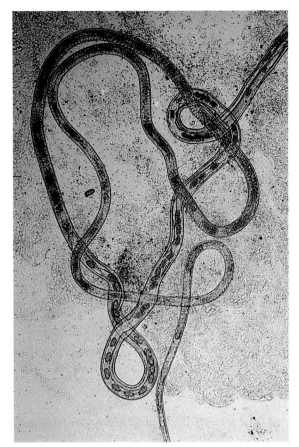

97. *Capillaria* spp. in a mount of gut contents. Length: 1-2 cm.

six months in the same aquarium were not infected. The worms live freely in the intestine and constantly wriggle. They have never been observed to hold fast by biting, hooking, or sucking onto the intestinal wall. The worms nourish themselves from the intestinal content and damage the host by removing nourishment from it. As with other nematodes, a mild infestation is well tolerated. If large numbers of worms appear, the fish become timid, darken, and eventually become emaciated. The female worms can attain a length of 4 millimeters, the males about 2 millimeters (Photograph No. 98). Adult females contain large numbers of eggs. Discharged eggs remain hanging together from the mother by long sticky threads. In massive infestations the threads gnarl together and form a sticky felt plug of eggs and worms that sticks in the intestine and may cause intestinal occlusion. The eggs develop rapidly, and the larvae hatch after only a few hours (Photograph No. 21, Chart 8). Transmission occurs through the eggs and larvae, which are eliminated in the feces and stay at the bottom until they are ingested by other fish feeding there.

More often it gets into the aquarium via infected new arrivals. Prevention consists of quarantining new fish and carrying out several microscopic examinations of feces during this time. Treatment according to method B_3 provides control for quite some time. Treatment with method C_5 has been used successfully. The only definitive treatment to annihilate the intestinal nematodes is with flubenol 5% (method C_6), since this also destroys the worms eggs.

7.5.2. Oxyurida (Pinworms or Threadworms)

Several years ago a new nematode species spread to the discus breeding facilities in the Rhein/Main region. The worms live mainly in the anterior area of the intestine. Up to now they have been demonstrated only in discus. Characids, gouramis, and cichlids that came into contact with infected discus for more than

98. Female threadworm of the order Oxyurida. Bright-field photograph. Size: 0.5-4mm.

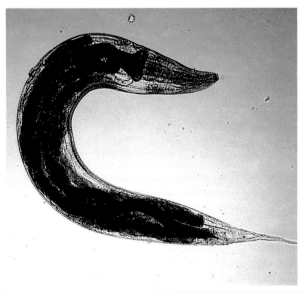

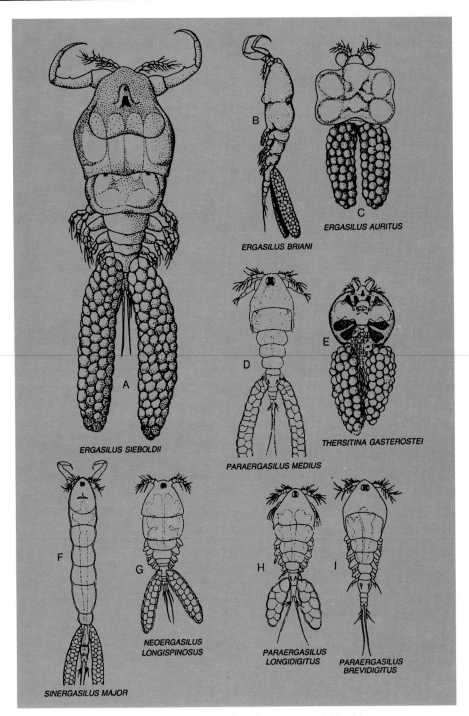

101: The family Ergasilidae; after Schäperclaus' *Fischk-rankheiten.*
a. *Ergasilus sieboldii* (about 1.7 mm); b. *Ergasilus briani* (Size: 0.7 - 1 mm); c. *Ergasilus auritus.* d. *Paraergasilus medius.* e. *Thersitina gasterostei;* f. *Sinergasilus major* (Size: 2.2 - 3.0 mm); g. *Neoergasilus longispinosus* (Size about 0.8 mm); h. *Paraergasilus longidigitus* (Size: 0.4 - 0.5 mm); i. *Paraergasilus brevidigitus.*

Chapter 8
ARTHROPODS

Arthropods parasitic on fish are rarely a problem in the aquarium. They are mainly crustaceans that live as parasites. Mites have not yet been definitely identified as parasites, although damage they have caused has been observed in aquarium fish.

8.1. Copepods

Copepods are dangerous to our fish for two reasons: there are several species that directly parasitize fish, and even harmless species can transmit dangerous worm diseases (Chapter 7.4 and 7.5.4). It is usually only the females that parasitize fish. They possess special clamping hooks to hold on to the fish, and their mouthparts are designed to suck the blood of the host. Many species have adapted so radically to this kind of life during the course of their evolution that they are difficult to recognize as crustaceans. A heavy infestation severely interferes with the fish's normal behavior. Methods C_7, C_{11}, and C_{18} can be applied to control the parasites.

8.1.1. Ergasilidae

In *Ergasilus* species, only the female is parasitic. They can be recognized by their elongated egg sacs and clasping hooks (Photograph No. 101). They are about 1.5 mm long. The egg sacs are scarcely a millimeter long and together can contain 50 to 200 eggs. There is only slight risk of introducing this parasite into the aquarium because only males are among the plankton in the water. It is, however, not impossible that females might be introduced as nauplii into the aquarium along with live foods. They will only reproduce, however, if sexually mature adults of both sexes are in the aquarium simultaneously or if fertilized females are introduced along with new fish.

Gill infestation is apparent to the naked eye. Crustacean parasites of the gills look like whitish, elongated objects on the gill filaments. They damage the fish by digesting its epithelial cells. Since they often change position on the fish, the gills suffer widespread damage.

Secondary infections often occur, particularly with fungus, which easily attacks the damaged tissues. Heavily infected fish suffer from anemia, become emaciated, and are susceptible to many other diseases. For that reason, no live food from fish ponds should be used. Treatment can be according to method C_{18a}, C_{11}, or C_7.

Besides the Ergasilidae, there are other copepods that parasitize freshwater and marine fish. Some attack the gill and buccal cavities as well as the skin of fish. Others cause boil-like growths on the head, in which the worm-like crustacean lives.

8.1.2. Lernaeide or Anchorworms

These very elongated copepods have lost their articulated appearance and thus resemble a worm more than they do a crustacean. On the head are amorphously shaped growths of chitin that serve to attach the parasite to the tissue of a fish (Photograph No. 102). Antennae and mouthparts are atrophied. The long, tube-like egg sacs are often rolled and twisted, not straight. *Lernaea* species and their relatives, the Lernaeopodidae, attack marine and freshwater fish. Depending upon the species, they live on the gills, in the gill and buccal cavities, on the skin and eyes, or in the musculature of the fish. The presence of these parasites in an aquarium is extremely rare. The control of parasites introduced along with fish can be carried out with method C_{12}, C_{18a}, C_{11}, or C_7.

8.2. Argulidae or Fish Lice

Fish lice are shield-shaped crustaceans that measure between 4 and 12 millimeters (Photograph No. 103). On the ventral surface are the eyes, sucking discs, two antennae with clasping hooks, and a spicule or sting with which the animal punctures the skin and sucks blood. The toxic substance injected by the louse when puncturing the skin can kill small fish, and in large fish the site of injection often becomes inflamed and swollen. The puncture wound can be secondarily infected by fungus;

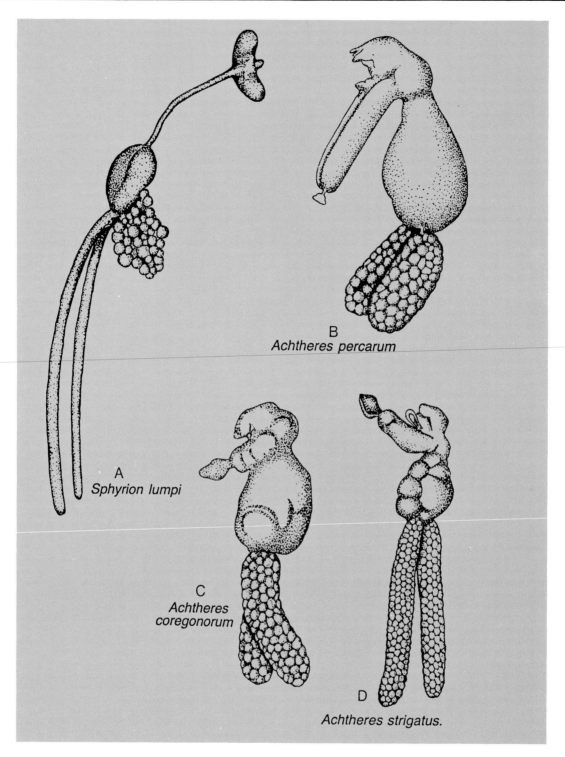

B
Achtheres percarum

A
Sphyrion lumpi

C
Achtheres coregonorum

D
Achtheres strigatus.

102 The Order Lernaeoidea, after Schäperclaus' *Fischkrankheiten.*
a. Sphyrion lumpi; b. Achtheres percarum; c. Achtheres coregonorum; d. Achtheres strigatus.

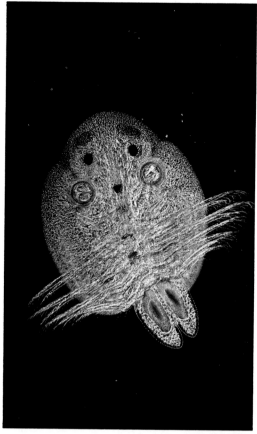

103. *Argulus* spp, carp louse. Bright field photograph. Size: 5-12mm.

it can also allow entry of the causative agent of abdominal dropsy and of blood parasites (see Chapters 4.2 and 6.1.1.).

After taking its meal, the parasite abandons the fish and swims freely around to find a new victim. If none is found, the parasite can survive three weeks without food.

Fish lice attack all fish species. They gain entry to the aquarium along with live foods from fish ponds or other bodies of water containing fish. Control of the parasites is possible with methods C_{12}, C_{18a}, C_{11}, and C_7.

8.3. Acarina or Fish Mites

Mites are not really fish parasites. Freshwater mites and their larval stages are predatory and can endanger the smallest fry. Since they occur in great numbers in ponds used for obtaining live foods, they are easily captured along with the live food and introduced with it into an aquarium. They do not reproduce if suitable food is lacking.

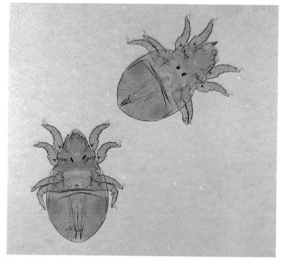

104. *Trimalaconothrus* spp. Mites mounted with E3. Size: 580u.

A species of mite recently has been spreading mostly among German discus-breeding facilities. Professor Beck of Karlsruhe has identified as a species of the genus *Trimalaconothrus* (Photograph No. 104). It usually is harmless, feeding on algae, debris, and fungal hyphae, but when food is extremely scarce for several weeks these mites climb up on fish and feed on their skin (Photograph No. 105). Massive infestations can endanger the fish, but only those which remain on the bottom at night. Infections of discus have never been observed. The mites are very resistant to chemical agents and high temperatures, and the only sure method to eliminate them is by drying out the tank. Since they eat debris and algae, however, they can be tolerated in the aquarium if kept under control.

105. *Trimalaconothrus* mites on the skin of a fish.

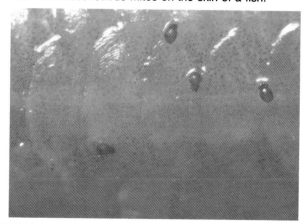

Chapter 9

DISEASES NOT CAUSED BY SPECIFIC PATHOGENIC ORGANISMS

The diseases discussed up to now were all caused by pathogens. There are also pathologic changes due to environmental factors (such as toxicity) or heredity. When environmental factors are the cause, normality is reestablished when the cause is removed, if the period of imbalance was not extended. It usually is too difficult to locate the cause, especially if it involves malnutrition and vitamin deficiencies, in which case the effects show up only after a long period. Sometimes the only evidence of deficiencies is the multiplication of certain parasites because they are taking advantage of the weakened resistance of the fish. Correction of the deficiency leads to improvement, but usually only after a long while.

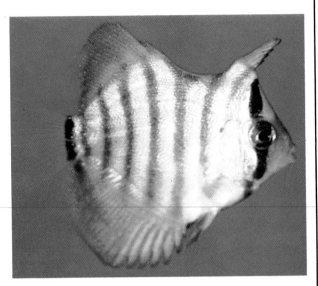

107. Fin deformation caused by deficiency during early growth phase.

9.1. Tumors and Growths

Tumors arise by uncontrolled division of somatic cells. These growths are neoplastic (i.e., new, abnormal, separate tissues taking nourishment from the body). There are various causes for them, usually chemicals (carcinogens) that stimulate individual cells to grow and proliferate uncontrollably. Moreover, predisposition to tumors may be inherited or caused by hormonal disorders. Tumors are classified as benign or malignant. The benign ones grow slowly, only push aside the adjacent tissues, and do not give rise to any daughter growths. Malignant tumors, however, grow fast and destroy adjacent tissues; they send cells through the bloodstream to other parts of the body and give rise to daughter growths or metastases at other locations.

Many tumors are caused by the effect of viruses or by aflatoxins (Chapter 9.3). Tumors generally do not occur very often in aquarium fish.

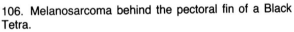

106. Melanosarcoma behind the pectoral fin of a Black Tetra.

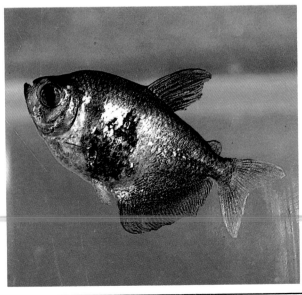

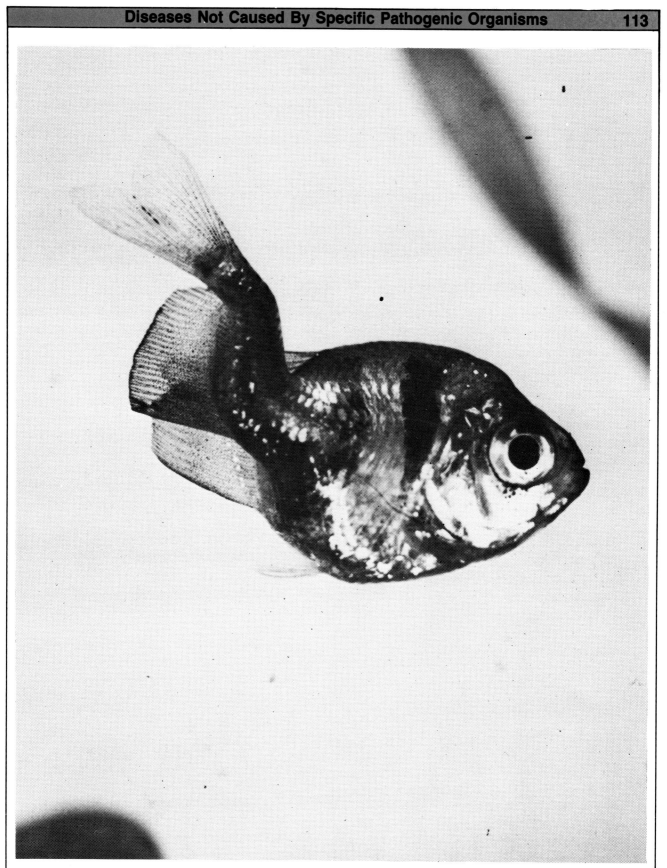

Obvious misshaping of aquarium fish can result from a number of different causes, with environmental and genetic factors both playing a part. In most cases it is not easy to pinpoint the exact cause of a deformation without having a good knowledge of the history of the affected specimen.

Thyroid tumors may be benign or malignant. They can be recognized at an early stage by a lifted operculum even while the fish is breathing calmly (Photograph No. 5, Chart 4). If the tumor is caused by iodine deficiency (goiter), then the addition of iodine to the aquarium water may cure the disease (method C_{10}). Malignant tumors (thyroid carcinomas) soon grow back if the diseased tissue is not completely excised. Metastases often appear in the same organ as well as sometimes in distant parts of the body. Treatment is impossible.

Lesions that arise from pigment cells (melanocytes or chromatophores) are called melanomas and melanosarcomas (Photograph No. 106). Their occurrence in livebearing species is often genetically determined and also can be purposely produced by hybridization (Photograph No. 6, Chart 4).

Lipomas are formed from fat cells (lipocytes or adipose cells) in the fatty tissue and can attain considerable size. These benign tumors are firm and can be removed whole from the surrounding tissues. A squash mount of a tumor fragment often squeezes out liquid fat in the form of small spheres.

Cysts form around foreign bodies and encapsulate them, isolating them from the other tissues. Parasites can likewise be enclosed in cysts. The hard bristles of various food animals, if they penetrate the intestinal wall, are often encapsulated as cysts (Photograph No. 28, Chart 14).

Cystomas are cysts that originate from the organs of the fish without any outside influence. The gallbladder, kidney, and air bladder are the organs usually affected. Cystomas attain considerable size and are filled with a turbid liquid. Externally, there is possible confusion with abdominal dropsy. This tumor is not treatable. Affected fish have to be sacrificed. When frequent tumors occur, check whether the water contains carcinogenic substances.

9.2. Malformations and Deformations

Malformations sometimes are seen in fish bred in the aquarium. Since this can be due to hereditary, such fish should not be bred further. If malformations show up often, then check to see whether all chemical factors in the environment are proper and that no vitamin deficiency is present. Fin deformations (Photograph No. 107) can be due to oxygen depletion, wrong pH, or vitamin deficiency. Shortened opercula result from vitamin and calcium deficiencies during growth (Photograph No. 1, Chart 1). Supplemental vitamins with Calcipot D_3 in the feed are a remedy, according to methods B_4, B_5, and C_{27} (Chapter 10).

Siamese twins, in which one sibling is present only as a knob or growth hanging from the belly of the other, is caused by damage (chemical or physical) to the egg. Other common anomalies are double organs, color aberrations, misshapen scales, skeletal deformations from vitamin deficiencies, eyes of unequal size, and dislocated lateral-lines.

9.3. Nutritional Problems

The importance of a balanced diet for the health of fish is still underestimated, even today. A one-sided diet can lead to signs of deficiencies, or at least to a reduced resistance to disease. Many dietary vitamins can be absorbed only if essential fats are present at the same time; otherwise these vitamins cannot

Malformations and deformations usually have a deleterious effect on the appearance of the fish and in most cases affect the fish's manueverability to some extent, but in some cases such anomalies are considered desirable and are actively perpetuated in aquarium-bred stock. The tailless cichlids shown here are not in the "desirable" category.

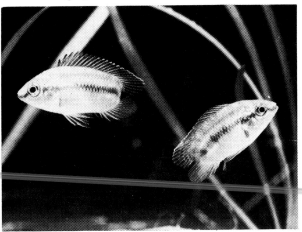

be utilized and are eliminated in the feces. It is important to know that beef-heart alone can never be adequate as food, but must be fed along with supplemental greens and occasionally with vitamins. The preparation of vitaminized feed is described in methods B_4 and B_5, Chapter 10.2. Several varied feedings with fresh or frozen live food daily are necessary. Aquarists who believe they have to give high vitamin doses should realize that too much of a good thing can be harmful. Constant overfeeding with vitamins, as well as not enough of them, can lead to disease. Vitaminized feed prepared according to method B_4 should not be given more than twice a week.

Bear in mind that more than two-thirds of the diseased fish examined in recent years exhibited major fatty degeneration of the liver and body cavity. Fatty degeneration leads to various disorders, including disrupted liver function (Photographs Nos. 48 and 49), often resulting in tuberculosis of the liver, spleen, and intestine. Also, the multiplication of various bacterial species in the liver, spleen, kidney, and body cavity can cause the signs of abdominal dropsy. Other parasites may multiply heavily because the resistance of the fish is reduced. Fatty degeneration of the liver is caused by too many carbohydrates and fats in the diet, as well as the lack of choline and vitamins. A one-sided diet with easily digestible feed, along with vitamin deficiency, leads to gastrointestinal inflammations. Spoiled feed is just as dangerous. Dry feed is worthless two months after the can is opened. Atmospheric humidity decomposes vitamins, giving bacteria and fungi a foothold. Moldy dry food must not, under any circumstances, be fed to the fish; the aflatoxins in it are highly toxic—5 mg aflatoxin per 1 kg of fish kills within a few days. The liver yellows and disintegrates (necrosis). Smaller concentrations of the toxin lead to liver cancer. It makes more sense to buy flake food in a can of just the right size to last at most six weeks.

According to experiences gathered over recent years, hole-in-the-head disease of the cichlids appears to be a deficiency disease that can have two causes. Up to now it has been ascribed to the flagellates *Hexamita* or,

in discus, *Spironucleus*. Cichlids have often been found with holes in the head area, yet their intestines were free of any flagellates. The flagellates found in the holes were often of nonparasitic species normally inhabiting aquarium water. In many instances, after successful control of the flagellates found along with hole-in-the-head disease, no improvement occurred in the fish with the disease.

On the other hand, holes in the head have been cleared up, even in the presence of flagellates, by the addition Osspulvit or Calcipot D_3.

These results lead to the conclusion that the occurrence of holes in the head and fins is a symptom of calcium, phosphorous, and vitamin D deficiencies in the diet. These substances are lacking in one-sided diets. In another case they were depleted in the intestine because of heavy (nonparasitic) flagellate infestation. The addition of vitamin powder according to method B_4 (Chapter 10) prevents hole-in-the-head disease.

Gastroenteritis (also called gastrointestinal inflammation) may result from spoiled feed, a vitamin deficiency, or a one-sided diet of meat (such as beef-heart). Likewise, a diet of an easily digestible food (such as white worms) with high nutritive value or a one-sided diet of carbohydrates, fats, or proteins can lead to the condition.

In one case, because of a lack of time, beef-heart without supplements was fed exclusively for two months to a tank of discus. That led to enteritis in four of the 16 discus, resulting in intestinal occlusion, whereby a 4-cm stretch of intestine became 2 cm thick, filled with half-digested food (Photograph No. 25, Chart ·11); the fish died with a severely bloated belly. A fourth fish recovered following a temperature increase to 33°C and administration of Osspulvit and spinach. Here, too, a clearly bloated belly was evident. Incompletely thawed frozen feed also causes enteritis.

9.4. Wounds

Skin abrasions, puncture wounds, and cuts sometimes are self-inflicted as frightened aquarium fish dart about. In combat with rival fish, it is not rare for the subordinate fish to sustain heavy skin damage. Pathogens then enter and cause infections, inflaming the wound or opening the way to fungal infections. Wounded fish must be transferred immediately to the quarantine tank. Treatment is with method C_{12}, C_{17d}, C_1, A_4, or C_{23}.

9.5. Diseases Caused by Chemicals

9.5.1. Oxygen Deficiency

There are various causes for oxygen deficiency in the aquarium, such as heavy feeding, overpopulation, poor aeration, dirty filters, and mulm-laden bottoms, for all decomposition processes burn up oxygen. Repeated bouts of oxygen deficiency can cause malformed young fish (Chapter 9.2). In oxygen-deficient water, the fish hang just under the surface of the water and breathe heavily. Dead fish lie in the tank, gills pale, the mouth and opercula open. If the fish show symptoms of a lack of oxygen, do not turn up the aeration excessively, for that only whips up any bottom mulm and causes even more oxygen loss. Therefore, regulate the aeration so it does not disturb the bottom matter and add hydrogen peroxide to the water (method C_{29}). If this does not improve the situation within a few minutes, then the fish are suffering from a gill disease (Chapter 3.4).

9.5.2. Acidosis and Alkalosis

Most fish are adapted to a stable pH value of 7, but it can vary between pH6 and pH8, depending upon species. As acidic pH values drop below 5.3, the fish begin to breathe heavier, dart backward through the aquarium, and gasp for air just under the surface of the water. Many tropical species live in extremely pure water that contains a large amount of humic acids, and these fish can tolerate distinctly lower pH values. At a stable, very slightly lowered pH value, a brown gill coating, mucous secretions on the gills, whitish skin opacities, or turbidity appears.

Alkalosis occurs when the pH value exceeds 8 by too much. The fish react with whitish skin turbidity and frayed fins, followed later by skin and gill corrosion or fraying. Ammonia toxicity also is a possibility.

9.5.3. Poisoning

Ammonia (NH_3) is strongly toxic to all fish. At a pH of under 7, it occurs as non-toxic ammonium (NH_4^+). An increase in pH (such as when carbon dioxide is taken up by plants under strong illumination) causes formation of free ammonia. Ammonium does not change at once to ammonia when the neutral pH value is exceeded, but depends upon the temperature at every pH value in a fixed percentage distribution. Thus, for example, at an ammonium content of 6-8 mg/l, a dangerous level of ammonia is reached only above pH 8. However, very small quantities of this substance suffice to considerably stress the fish. A balanced aquarium with a well run-in filter is hardly in danger, since ammonium is metabolized by bacteria and very little of it is present.

Ammonia poisoning shows up at a level of more than 0.3 mg/l as skin and nerve damage. Hemorrhages next appear first on the gills then on the epidermis and internal organs. Drop the pH to below 7 to achieve rapid improvement. Chemical tests for ammonia are available commercially. From the foregoing, it is obvious that the use of such tests makes sense only along with pH measurements.

Nitrite and nitrate are the oxidation products of ammonia. They form as a result of high levels of ammonium following heavy organic pollution of the water (such as following overfeeding). If nitrites accumulate in the water without oxidizing into nitrates, the toxicity that occurs can be fatal to the fish. They become apathetic and die suddenly in full color.

Sometimes nitrites occur along with oxygen depletion. Nitrates are not as toxic as nitrites and are tolerated at much higer levels. To prevent accumulation, water must be changed regularly or else gradually exchanged out of the aquarium. An excessively high nitrite level can be lowered only by repeated water changes. Nitrite toxicity for fish starts at 10 mg/l. Nitrate toxicity starts at 100 to 300 mg/l.

If the filter motor ever fails, an oxygen deficit occurs rapidly in the closed filter chamber. The filter organisms, normally bathed in oxygen-rich water, die. A stinking soup of by-products of anaerobic reactions forms and produces large quantities of nitrites. When the motor starts up again, this toxin-laden water will be pumped out into the aquarium water, and in a short time the fish will show signs of poisoning that can be fatal. One hour can be taken as the limit of inactivity if the filter is not too dirty. If, however, the power outage lasts longer, then the filter must be throughly cleaned before starting it up again.

Carbon dioxide (CO_2) dissolves more easily than oxygen in water, thus carbon-dioxide fertilized aquariums could accumulate dangerous levels if the metering dispenser malfunctions. It is completely irrational to give carbon dioxide at night, for then the plants do not use it. In the absence of light no oxygen is produced, letting the CO_2 level rise. The fish react with difficult breathing, greatly increased respiratory rate, restless swimming around, rolling or reeling, assuming of diagonal or horizontal positions on the bottom for short periods, loss of reflexes, respiratory failure, and death. Strong aeration drives off the carbon dioxide, but only very slowly; it is better to change a large portion of the water.

Hydrogen sulfide is generated (anaerobically) by decomposition in the bottom matter. Hydrogen sulfide consumes the free oxygen in the water, leading to symptoms of suffocation and intoxication. The gills turn violet-red and hemorrhages appear.

Chemical substances from outside the aquarium can poison fish, too. To avoid fish mortality, do not let the aquarium air pump suck up any organic solvents, aerosols from spray paints or insecticides, or fumes from oil heaters and furnaces. Some roots, pebbles, plastics, and colored decorative items can liberate toxic substances into the water.

Chlorine toxicity causes shakiness in movement and pale fins. Later, the fish turn dull and stop breathing. Remove the chlorine from tap water before adding it to the aquarium. Chemicals can be used, the water can be allowed to sit in an open container, the water can be heated and then cooled, or the water can be run through a shower-head arrangement to release the chlorine.

Misuse of medications can cause toxicity. The fish turn pale, are timid and hide, and may also shoot madly through the aquarium. If these symptoms appear after administration of medication, quickly replace a large portion of the water. Since the toleration of a medication varies from species to species, a new one first must be tested. Heed the dosage instructions closely.

Copper toxicity may occur in treatments with copper sulfate if the water hardness is not at least 10°DH. It may likewise occur if the water comes through copper tubing. Let it run awhile first. Herbicides for algae also contain copper and should not be overused. Rapid changes of water are the only countermeasures that can be recommended. Iron in fertilizer and lead wires on plants can lead to toxicity. Regular addition of Fetrilon is said to lead to liver damage, though this is not experimentally demonstrated.

9.6. Gas Bubble Disease

Just as in divers who ascend too rapidly, gas bubbles form in the fins and skin of fish when there is a sudden reduction in gas (air) pressure. The bubbles are quite visible to the naked eye and the skin crackles if you run your finger over it. In extreme cases, gas bubbles in the blood kill the fish (gas embolus). Gas pressure can be lowered by changing large portions of the water, sudden lowering of the temperature, and by exposing thickly planted landscapes to sunshine. Gas bubbles also can form when fish are moved without first slowly exchanging travel water with aquarium water. Gas bubble disease cannot occur in a well-aerated aquarium.

9.7. Injury Caused by Temperature

Water temperature represents for the fish one of the most important environmental factors, so the temperatures reported in the literature should be adhered to as closely as possible. Species of fish whose optimal temperatures are more than 4°C apart should not be in the same aquarium community.

Digestion and the functioning of the internal organs depend directly upon the water temperature. For that reason, sudden changes in temperature are very bad for the whole organism. An aquarist can make the greatest mistake by dumping the fish from the transport bag into the aquarium without first having equalized the temperatures. Sudden increases in temperature have as negative an effect as drops in temperature.

Adaptation of the fish to temperature should be slow, not exceeding about 1°C per hour. Temperature changes should be utilized only in the treatment of diseases. Even then, the fluctuation should not be more than 1°C per hour. Many fish live in waters where temperatures fluctuate sharply, such as dropping several degrees at night. Whoever cares for such fish under natural conditions and wants them to multiply should relaize that they cannot be fed in the evening under any condition. A drop in temperature greatly slows down digestion, thus leaving undigested food in the intestine, resulting in enteritis, followed later by infections caused by diseases associated with weakness.

Sharp rises or drops in temperature because of faulty thermostats may be harmless if the change takes several hours to occur. The fish die only when the aquarist changes a large quantity of water, changing the proper temperature too rapidly.

Chapter 10

TREATMENT OF DISEASED FISH

10.1. General Guidelines for Medication

The relatively small amount of water in a tank is a considerable disadvantage for the health of fish but is an advantage in treating them. In the first place, the quantity of water is precisely measurable, so that the exact dosage with the best spectrum of action can be given. In the second place, just minute quantities of very expensive drugs may be involved.

Most drugs and other chemicals used in the control of fish diseases are toxic, and they must be kept away from children.

The effect of therapeutic chemicals and pigments is based upon their being more toxic to parasites than to the host. The greater the difference in toxicity, the safer the medication. Unfortunately, however, the limits of tolerance for fish and parasite toward the best drugs are often quite similar, so dosage instructions (quantity and dosage schedule) must be strictly adhered to. In addition, the drug's effect and the fish's tolerance to it are closely dependent upon the quality and temperature of the water; the tolerance varies from species to species. Underdosage is as a rule to be avoided, since no parasites will be killed. Preventive treatment on a constant or regular basis also is irrational, indeed even dangerous. Such a procedure leads to the development of resistant parasites that then cannot be controlled even with higher dosages.

Since parasites also have optimal temperatures at which they can reproduce best, there is the possibility of backing up drug therapy with temperature adjustment. Outside of their optimal temperature, the parasites are often more susceptible to the drug. Whether the temperature should be turned up or down depends upon the drug. Sometimes the toxicity rises with the temperature (e.g., Masoten, method C_{18}). Temperature instructions for medications, therefore, must be strictly followed.

In general, when treating with a certain medication a species of fish with which you do not have any experience, you cannot predict anything about tolerance. It is absolutely essential to carry out a therapeutic trial with a single, severely affected fish. Select the weakest one. If it tolerates the treatment, others of the same species can also be treated. Pay particular attention to catfish and characins in community tanks—these groups of fishes are especially sensitive to many medication side-effects.

Some kinds of treatment should be done in the fully setup aquarium so as to hit the pathogens that are not the fish itself. Other treatments are carried out in separate containers, otherwise the bacterial flora of the filter and the bottom of the aquarium will be killed, thus leading to the formation of toxins in the water. Many medications contain vehicles that can cause a huge increase in bacteria and oxygen consumption (e.g., Gabbrocol, method C_8) and so cannot be administered to fish in a setup aquarium.

The method of administration for every drug and the length of time to let it act are spelled out in the instructions. Yet it is possible that weakened or sensitive fish still may not tolerate the dosage. Even antibiotic therapy does not always immediately stop fish from dying, especially in bacterial infections that damage internal organs; individuals die of the disease even following successful treatment because damaged internal organs cease functioning.

As a rule, fish are treated in a long bath in the aquarium for one to several days. You can readily understand that drugs that act against bacteria on the fish can also damage other bacteria and microorganisms elsewhere in the tank. Some die and pollute the water.

Since the filter also contains bacteria, it is better to first wash out the filter media. Activated charcoal must be removed before treatment begins. Change a good percentage of the water several times after the treatment. Replace a portion of the substrate in the filter with activated charcoal, which will remove the rest of the drug from the water. Following the use of many kinds of drugs, the filter needs several weeks to rebuild an active bacterial flora. Handling of the filter material is briefly described, when appropriate, in the section on methods of treatment. Ultraviolet light can decompose many water-soluble medications, so the UV lamps in the filtration system should be turned off during the course of treatment.

Short baths can last from a few minutes to hours and are carried out in small tanks containing an accurately measured volume of water. These baths are useful when a high dosage of the medication is required. The temperature and chemistry of the water must match those of the regular aquarium. Watch the fish closely during this short bath. If they turn on their sides, remove them from the bath at once. Never give short baths in the aquarium, for that would kill all plants and bacteria; it would be impossible to remove the drug fast enough. A pharmacist or veterinarian can help you obtain some of the medications, but a pet shop should have convenient dosage forms of many especially prepared for home aquarists.

The aquarist should become familiar with the standard weights and measures used in the preparation of solutions of medications and other chemicals. In the metric system, weight is given in grams (g) or milligrams (mg); 1 gram = 1000 milligrams. To measure liquids, the aquarist uses a beaker of known volume, a graduated cylinder, or measuring pipettes. Liquids in the metric system are measured by the liter (l or L) or milliliter (ml), or occasionally, cubic centimeter (cc or cm^3). One liter = 1000 ml or 1000 cc.

An accurate balance with a range of 0.5 to 50 grams is needed. Otherwise, a pharmacist might be willing to measure out the minute quantities you would need to give in a treatment. The pet shop, however, usually has dosages measured just for fish. At times the expense of buying expensive drugs in bulk can justify several aquarists pooling their resources.

Stock solutions are needed for many thera-peutic baths, which are made by dissolving a certain amount of drug in a liter of water. One milliliter of this mixture thus contains one-thousandth part of the whole amount. As a rule, one gram of drug is dissolved in one liter of water to make a stock solution, each milliliter of which contains one milligram of drug.

10.2 Therapeutic Recommendations

The following therapeutic recommendations are numbered to correspond with the diseases described in previous chapters. Quantities stated are tolerated by most fish species; treatments for catfishes, characins, and smaller cichlids, however, should first be tested as previously described.

Many drugs mentioned here are powerful chemicals used also in human medicine. They also can produce more serious side-effects than the pet shop products and should be used only after precise diagnoses and never without good reason. They should be used only when pet shop medications fail. Labels on pet shop medications should list contents and intended uses. There are no true "miracle" drugs, so be cautious about so-called cure-alls.

Two individually safe drugs can be dangerous if used together. Different diseases should be treated successively, with the more serious disease treated first. Allow a recuperation period of at least three days between treatments and clear the water of all medications by changing water, as described earlier, even if the same treatment is being repeated.

Wrong uses of antibiotics have led to resistant pathogens; the fear is that this resistance can be transferred to man's bacterial pathogens. Expert opinion varies widely, but antibiotics should be used in aquariums only in direst emergencies. Sulfonamides and nitrofurans should be tried first. Antibiotic therapy should be done in bare all-glass tanks; the antibiotic solutions must not be allowed into the sewer system. They should be left in the treatment tank and heated to between 50° and 60° C.; decomposition should occur within two days except for chloramphenicol, which can be destroyed in two hours through the addition of lye or caustic soda to raise the pH to over 10.

Mixing medications into the food is often recommended; the medication goes directly to the gut, and treatment can be given in a fully set up aquarium. Putting the medicine into the food of course requires that the fish is accustomed to the food and is not too sick to eat. (Refer to methods C_{27} and B_5.)

The medications listed below are not intended for use with food fish.

The following therapeutic recommendations have been thoroughly tested, but there is no guarantee how the medications will react in different waters. Some substances dissolved in the water can increase toxicity, while others can act bactericidally and destroy important bacteria, leading to poisoning of the tank and death of fish. Other medications can lead to bacterial overgrowth, which can cause water turbidity and symptoms of oxygen depletion in fish. Problems can often be avoided by changing the water and filters regularly.

Avoid giving medications to fish at night, because they should be observed for several hours after administering. If the fish show any signs of toxicity, change the water or transfer the fish to fresh water. In cases of oxygen depletion, install additional aeration.

Because of the above reasons, we cannot assume responsibility for the success or safety of these therapeutic recommendations.

10.3. Methods A-D
Method A_1
Chloramphenicol (Chloromycetin®)
Use: Abdominal dropsy, furunculosis, bacterial fin rot, vibriosis, bacterial gill disease.

Spectrum of action: Gram-positive bacteria, cocci, and spore bacilli; Gram-negative bacteria and cocci; actinomycetes, flexibacteria, spirochetes, rickettsias, and large viruses.

The drug can be stored, cool and dry, for years. Use as a long bath in a separate container.

Dosage: 40 mg per liter of water for 10 to 20 hours. The drug can be dissolved in a small quantity of ethyl alcohol before adding it to the treatment tank. During treatment, run the filter over clean absorbent or raw cotton or foam filter material. Check on the fish and the condition of the water often. If the water turns turbid, take the fish out and, if need be, transfer them to freshly mixed solution.

Chloramphenicol can be mixed into the feed according to method B_5. Since it tolerates temperatures up to 100°C, it can be stirred in at a temperature of 80°C.

Dosage in feed: 500 mg per 100 g feed, given twice daily for three days.

Method A_2
Combination treatment for *Columnaris* disease with chloramphenicol + acriflavin (trypaflavin)
Carry out treatment as in A_1.

Dosage: 4 ml stock solution of acriflavin (see method C_1) to a liter of aquarium water, to which is added 40 mg chloramphenicol per liter water. Length of treatment is 12 hours.

Method A_3
Neomycin sulfate
Use: External bacterial diseases such as fin rot, skin lesions, and the new discus disease.

Spectrum of action: Gram-negative bacteria and cocci. Administer as a long bath in a separate container and filter over clean raw cotton or foam filter material.

Dosage: 2 g to 100 liters of water for three days. In rare cases, sensitive fish can be poisoned.

Dosage in feed: 250 mg mixed into 100 g feed according to method B_5. Feed three times a day at four-hour intervals for three days. Maximal temperature when mixing is 40°C. This method is useless for infections of most internal organs and is used only for intestinal infections.

Combination with nitrofurantoin (see method C_{21}) at the above dosage can be effective in the new disease of discus. The precondition is that the usually present secondary parasites be controlled first. Transfer the fish to clean, freshly prepared water before treatment. The fish remain in the bath for three to five days, then they are transferred to fresh water. A follow-up treatment with nitrofurantoin can be carried out for six to ten days, but is usually not necessary.

Method A$_4$
Combisonum eye ointment containing neomycin (see A$_3$)

Combisonum is the drug of choice when fish have injured themselves. It protects against bacterial infection and fosters healing. Take the fish out of the aquarium (quarantine tank) every day and wrap it in a wet towel. Dry the wound carefully with blotter paper, which also removes any dead tissue. Then apply Combisonum. When the edges of the wound begin to close over, apply treatment only every second or third day. As prophylaxis, a fungicidal ointment can be applied every third day or a mycostatic agent added to the water (method C$_{12}$ or C$_{17d}$).

Method A$_5$
Tetracycline HCl
Use: Abdominal dropsy, vibriosis.

Spectrum of actions: Gram-positive cocci and bacteria, Gram-negative cocci, bacteria, actinomycetes, spirochetes, and large viruses.

This drug can be given as a permanent bath at Dosage A (see below) in an already setup aquarium, with filtration over clean raw cotton or foam filter material. The water becomes colored and several plant species will be damaged, so the use of a separate container is recommended.

Dosage A: 1 g to 100 liters of water for four days.

Dosage B: 100 mg per 1 liter of water for 24 hours (only in a separate container).

In the feed described under method B$_5$, 750 mg tetracyclin HCl is mixed with 100 g feed and then administered two times daily at six-hour intervals for seven days. Stir in at a temperature of 40°C.

Method A$_6$
Chlortetracyclin, Oxytetracyclin (contained in Aureomycin and Terramycin—Hen)
Use: Usage, effect, and dosage in regard to the tetracyclin content are equivalent to A$_5$. Because of the other ingredients in it, Terramycin is used only in feedstuffs.

Doxycycline 100 is likewise a tetracyclin. It is known as Vibramycin.

Dosage: The content of one capsule to 20 liters of water for two to four days.

Method B$_1$
Heat treatment

The raising of temperature as therapy has a long history. It should be raised slowly and not more than 1°C hourly. The rational of this therapy is to create an environment in which the pathogen is no longer viable or able to reproduce. Not all species of fish can tolerate higher temperatures. Chemical treatment is sometimes easier on the fish. Heat therapy can be applied for the following pathogens:

Costia spp.: 33°C for four days
Ichthyophthirius spp.: 33°C for ten days
Oodinium spp.: 33°-34°C for 24 to 36 hours.
Absolutely clean water and good aeration are essential.

If the fish do not seem to feel well and this is not due to polluted water or chemical causes, an increase in temperature of 3°C for two or three days can have a very positive effect. Resistance against infections is increased because more antibodies are formed. For discus the temperature can be raised even as high as 35°C. Greater increases in temperature, however, burden the fish's metabolism too severely, so that stress increases and resistance again drops.

Method B$_2$
Transfer method

With this method, the life cycle of *Ichthyophthirius* can be interrupted, thus preventing spread of the disease. The method takes time and effort, requiring five containers. Every 12 hours the fish are transferred to a new container. The cysts that drop off release their swarmer cells only after the fish have already been transferred to the next container. When the fish "recycle" on the sixth day to their first container, the swarmer cells have already died. The temperature in all containers should be 25°C. If the treatment lasts 23 days, you can be rather certain that the fish are free of "ich." The daily handling for transfer, however, stresses the fish quite severely.

Method B$_3$
Screening method

This method is appropriate for all parasites that do not develop any motile swarmer cells or larvae. It is used mainly in the breeding of schools of fish. In the breeding tanks, a screen or grid is installed at a height of 2 to 5 cm above the bottom. The mesh is too small for the fish, but allows the eggs of the parasites to fall through along with the fecal matter, thus dropping them out of the fish's reach. The emerging larvae die. The problem, however, is vacuuming out the mulm that collects under the screen.

Method B₄
Vitaminized feed

You can easily produce your own vitaminized feed that contains all the important vitamins and trace elements. Scrape some beef-heart onto a plate and add half as much of finely shredded deep-frozen spinach. Spread it all out into a layer about 3 to 5 mm thick. Then sprinkle enough vitamin powder over it until the whole surface is whitish (see also method C₂₇).

The use of liquid vitamins is ineffective because it does not adhere to the feed. Spread the same amount of brewer's yeast powder (from a health food store) evenly over the feed and leave it there until the beef-heart and spinach thaw out (about 15 minutes). Then mix it all together, kneading it well, and feed it right to the fish. Finely grated carrots can substitute for the spinach.

When using Osspulvit—N, Neocalcit tablets, and Calcipot D₃, vitamins missing from these products can be provided with VMP tablets (Pfizer) by pounding the tablets and sprinkling the powder, as described above, on the spread-out feed patty.

Method B₅
Recipe for preparation of medicinal feed

Prepare a mash of two-thirds beef-heart or lean beef and one-third spinach. Both ingredients must be minced small enough to be ingested by small fish. After thorough mixing, 50-gram portions are frozen in small plastic containers or bags then later thawed as needed.

Now, to a small tin can, add 50 ml cold water and 1 gram powdered agar agar. A tiny amount of red food dye makes the feed more appetizing, as does some Maggi (brand name of a German herbal or condiment additive for food seasoning), not more than needed for a cup of soup. Stir with a small fork while heating the can of mix in a water bath until the agar dissolves and the solution thickens. At about 80°C, stir in the 50g beef mash in small portions without letting the temperature drop significantly. When all the beef mash is stirred in, remove the tin can from the water bath and let it cool slowly. Depending upon its heat stability, the medication is stirred into the hot, liquid feed or added just before solidification at about 40-50°C (follow the instructions under methods of treatment). Many antibiotics do not tolerate any heat, so the feed must be cooled down quickly (in a refrigerator to 2-5°C) after stirring in the active ingredient. Do not let it freeze, or the agar again liquifies. The finished feed has a solid, rubbery consistency and fish like to eat it once they become accustomed to it. It can be kept three days in a refrigerator at 2 to 5°C.

For feeding, cut the mass into mouth-sized bits that will remain solid in the aquarium at up to a temperature of 28°C (just 82°F). After 12 hours at the most, all uneaten food must be removed from the tank, otherwise it will become moldy. Any antibiotics mixed into the feed soon lose their efficacy, therefore do not give more medicated feed than can be eaten in an hour.

Method C₁
Acriflavin (Trypaflavin)

Use: Skin turbidity or clouding, mouth rot, fin rot, and disinfection of small wounds.

Spectrum of action: *Costia* spp., *Chilodonella* spp., *Trichodina* spp., *Trichodinella* spp., flexibacteria, fin and skin turbidity or cloudiness.

Both names refer to the same drug. It dyes intensely. Acriflavin can be put into the completley set up aquarium but severely damages plants. The filter substrate should be cleaned before addition of the drug. After the treatment, filter over activated charcoal to remove the drug.

Stock Solution: 1 g to 1 liter of water.

Dosage A: 1 ml stock solution to each liter of aquarium water to prevent infections.

Dosage B: 3 ml stock solution to each liter of water for four days to help against infections in the early stage.

Dosage C: 5 ml stock solutions to each liter water in a separate container for two to four days against *Columnaris* spp., *Costia* spp., *Trichodina* spp., and *Chilodonella* spp.

Dosage D: 10 ml stock solution to each liter water in a separate container for 20 days (against *Ichthyophthirius* spp.) or for 10 days (against *Oodinium* spp.). **Caution:** *Many fish do not tolerate this dosage.*

Method C₂
Alcohol

Leeches attached to fish can be removed by pressing an alcohol-soaked cotton swab briefly on the leech. The fish must be lifted out of the water for this treatment.

Method C₃
Basic (or alkaline) brilliant green

This dye comes in various fish medication preparations available at pet shops, and these are more convenient to use than the pure brilliant green.

Use: Skin turbidity (or cloudiness), fin rot, gill rot, skin fungus, mouth fungus.

Spectrum of Action: Gram-positive bacteria, skin fungi, and protozoa.

Carry out the treatment in a separate tank, with the water filtered over clean absorbent cotton or foam filter material. **This treatment is toxic to many fish.**

Stock solution: 1 g to each liter water. Keep in a brown or amber bottle.

Dosage A: 2 ml stock solution to 12.5 liters water for 24 hours, then total change of water, or transfer the fish to another container. This treatment can be repeated on the third day. For bacterial infections of the skin.

Dosage B: 2 ml stock solution to 15 liters of water. Bathe the fish in this solution four hours at a time on three successive days. The working solution must be freshly made for every treatment (i.e., add stock solution to fresh water each time). Used for parasites and fungi.

Method C₄
Quinine sulfate, quinine HCl

Use: Freshwater *Oodinium.*

Dosage: 1 g quinine to 100 liters water as a continuous bath for three days.

Quinine poisons fish that are sensitive to it and lower animals do not tolerate it very well. Quinine HCl is preferred over quinine sulfate. Although quinine decomposes after some time in water, it is better to filter it out over activated charcoal after the treatment. Clean the filter substrate before treatment. It is safer to treat the fish in a separate small tank and then treat the aquarium by itself. That way no fish will die when the water is poured into the aquarium. Afterward, change all the water. Transfer the fish to separate treatment tanks containing freshly prepared medication if the aquarium water becomes turbid.

Method C₅
Concurat L 10%

This is a broad-spectrum vermifuge for cattle, sheep, goats, swine, and poultry. Because of its sweet taste, it must be kept out of the reach of children.

Use: Intestinal nematodes.

Dosage A: Dissolve 2 g Concurat in 1 liter of water. Soak living bloodworms in this solution until the first larvae die, then immediately feed the still living ones to the fish.

Dosage B: Mix 1 g Concurat into 100 g feed. Stir into feed made by method B₅ at 50°C. Give once daily over five days.

Method C₆
Flubendazol & acetone or DMSO, flubenol 5%

Flubendazol is a solvent used for gill, skin and intestinal worms. Since the active ingredient is insoluble in water, it has to be first dissolved in an organic solvent. Dimethylsulfoxide (DMSO) was used in recent years. It is very toxic and should not come in contact with unprotected human skin. In no case should children get hold of it. Fish tolerate it well when no other chemicals or drugs are in the water. Even water preparation substances can become toxic in the presence of DMSO. The tank or breeding facilities must be in an absolutely clean condition. High levels of nitrite or ammonia, in the presence of DMSO, can become lethal to fish.

Rinsing out the filter material and changing a large portion of the water beforehand has a good effect. DMSO also cause an unpleasant tank odor for weeks. Since treatment also kills gill worm eggs, the treatment does not have to be repeated. Because of all of the above risks associated with DMSO, it should not be used by aquarists any longer.

Acetone has been used very successfully since 1988 as a well tolerated solvent for flubendazol. All gill and intestinal worms as well as their eggs are destroyed. Only at 100x normal dosage does acetone become toxic to fish. It does not leave any unpleasant odors in the vicinity of the tank. Feeding with flubenol 5% in feed mix B5 destroys the intestinal worms, but re-infection is possible when fish pick up eggs from the bottom.

Dosage A: For each 100 liters tank water, put 200 mg flubenol 5% in a small glass (do not use plastic) and then add 5 ml acetone or DMSO. After agitating several minutes, distribute the milky suspension over the surface of the water. After five to eight days begin to remove the medication by water changes. The water can become slightly turbid. Aerate the water well during treatment. Bacterial overgrowth may occur in many cases, causing turbidity and oxygen-depletion sysmptoms in the fish. An immediate major water change is necessary.

Dosage B: Add 100 mg flubenol 5% to 100g feed mix B5. Give it five times every second day. On those days feed only once with the regular diet.

Microscopic monitoring of the treatment will not reveal any results for ten days, but after this time the worms begin to die. That is expected because flubenol 5% blocks the resorption of certain nutrients from the intestine, thus starving the worms. That takes about eight days for gill worms, for Oxyurida about ten days, and for *Capillaria* about 15 days. In the female worms, however, damage to the egg walls can be seen as soon as the second day of treatment. They seem malformed and burst when expelled. Therefore there are no worm eggs visible in the feces or on the gills by the third day of treatment.

Method C₇
Formalin (35 to 45% solutions of formaldehyde)

Formalin is highly toxic and carcinogenic.

Use: Ectoparasites on skin and gills. Do not use if the fish have large-area skin wounds *(Costia* and "ich" in advanced stage).

Spectrum of action: Gill and skin worms, *Chilodonella* spp., *Trichodina* spp.

Dosage; Short bath with 2 to 4 ml formalin in 10 liters of water for 30 minutes in a separate tank.

Observe the fish well. Stop treatment if the fish lose equilibrium. Many fish tolerate formalin very poorly. For egg-laying gill worms, the treatment can be repeated in three days. After treatment, transfer the fish to a parasite-free tank. For *Brooklynella hostilis,* Blasiola recommends 2.6 ml formalin to 10 liters of seawater in a separate tank.

Method C₈
Gabbrocol

Use: White, slimy feces.

Spectrum of action: Intestinal flagellates and ciliates.

Gabbrocol has proven itself against flagellates and ciliates. It can be used as a long bath or in the feed made by method B₅.

A Gabbrocal bath is problematical because the vehicle that carries the active ingredient is glucose. Treatment must take place only in an empty glass tank with vigorous aeration and filtration over clean absorbent cotton or foam filter material. Glucose causes heavy turbidity in the water because of bacterial reproduction. After about 18 hours an oxygen deficiency often occurs, causing the fish to have difficulty breathing and then suffocating. For that reason even robust fish should not, as a rule, remain longer than 18 hours in the solution.

The fish must be transferred to clean water, at the latest when the bath water becomes turbid. This amount of time is adequate for the treatment. If you want to be extra certain, then transfer the fish after 12 hours to another aquarium containing freshly added Gabbrocol solution. Bacterial proliferation and thus water turbidity can be delayed by using distilled water or boiled tap water. The treatment tanks must be thoroughly washed out with hot water.

Dosage: Dissolve 5 g Gabbrocol (one bag) in 30 liters of water. Let the fish bathe in this for 18 hours. In severe cases, the bath can be repeated in another tank containing freshly added solution.

Dosage in feed: Mix 2 g Gabbrocol into 100 g feed (see method B_5) at 40°C and feed for three days. In severe cases, feed the mix until the white feces disappear, at which point continue the treatment for another three days.

Method C_9
Griseofulvin, Fulvicin tablets (500 mg)
Use: Mouth fungus, skin fungus, gill rot, and other mycoses.

Spectrum of action: Almost all external fungi on fish.

Since usually only a few fish are affected, prepare the long bath in a separate tank.

Dosage: 10 mg to 1 liter, or a 500 mg tablet in 50 liters of water.

Pound the tablets into powder and pre-dissolve in some warm water. Three days after the hyphae disappear, the treatment can be stopped. If the aquarium is already set up, this treatment may damage the plants. After treatment, change half of the water and filter out the rest of the drug over activated charcoal.

Method C_{10}
Potassium iodide and iodine
Use: Thyroid swelling.

Benign thyroid tumors can be treated with these chemicals, showing improvement only after two to four weeks, at which time the swelling or tumor slowly regresses. Carry out the treatment in the aquarium. Do not filter over charcoal.

Stock solution: 0.5 g iodine and 5 g potassium iodide dissolved in 100 ml water.

Dosage: With a pipette, add 1 drop of the stock solution to every 5 liters of aquarium water. More precisely, add 1 ml stock solution to 50 liters of aquarium water. The appropriate dosage is re-added after every water change.

Method C_{11}
Potassium permanganate
Use: Very heavy infestation with the parasites listed below.

Spectrum action: *Trichodina* spp., *Argulus* spp., gill worms, *Saprolegnia* spp.

Treat the fish with a short (immersion) bath of 30-45 seconds in a separate container. The dosage that causes toxicity is close to the level needed to kill the parasites, so this treatment should be used only for emergencies. Treatment according to method C_{18} is easier on the fish. The effect of medication is significantly weaker in organically polluted water than it is in clean water.

Dosage: Short (immersion) bath of 100 mg potassium permanganate to 10 liters of water. Monitor the fish closely during the bath. For gill worms, repeat the bath on the third day. Do not return the fish to the contaminated (or infested) tank before it is disinfected (see method C_{18}).

Continuous treatment with small amounts of potassium permanganate for a few hours or days is irrational, since it is not stable in water.

Method C_{12}
NaCl (kitchen, rock, mineral, or sea salt)
Salt is most certainly the oldest medication used in fish diseases.

Use: Incipient skin and fin cloudiness (or turbidity) and mild infestation with the parasites listed below.

Spectrum of action: *Costia* spp., *Chilodonella* spp., *Trichodina* spp., fungi, leeches.

For mild cases, salt is used in long and short baths.

Dosage A: (short bath): 15-20 g for each liter of water. Bath lasts 10 to 45 minutes.

Dosage B : (long bath): 1 g to each 12.5 liters of water in the aquarium for soft-water fish. 3 g to each 10 liters of water for hard-water fish. Intermediate values have to be estimated. After five days, the salt content can be reduced by changing the water.

Plants can be damaged starting at a salt concentration of 2 grams per 10 liters of aquarium water.

We can prepare our own physiological saline for microscopy by dissolving 6.4 g of salt in 1 liter of water. Its use is explained in Chapter 11.

Method C₁₃

Copper sulfate, CuSo₄·5 H₂O (blue crystals)
Use: *Oodinium,* algae, fungi, and mixed infections with the following listed below.
Spectrum of action: *Costia* spp., *Saprolegnia* spp., *Branchiomyces, Oodinium,* algae, and *Gyrodactylus.*
Stock solution: 1 g copper sulfate and 0.25 g citric acid to 1 liter of distilled water.
Dosage: 12.5 ml to 10 liters of aquarium water for ten days. Administer half of this on days three, five, and seven.

Test reagents for copper have been available for some time now among the diagnostic sets for water chemistry. During treatment, the copper content of the water should not drop below 0.12 mg/L and not rise over 0.18 mg/L (using the Aqua Merck copper test no. 14651, Duplatest CU). Test every other day and add any missing coopper (1 ml stock solution = 1 mg CuSO₄). Lower animals do not tolerate the treatment. They must either be removed from the aquarium until the copper level again drops below 0.3 mg/L, or else the fish must be transferred to a spacious glass tank and treated there. Filter over clean cotton or foam filter material. For fungi and algae, the affected fish can be treated in a short bath of 1 gram of copper sulfate to 10 liters of water for 10 to 20 minutes. Plants may be damaged. Freshwater must first be hardened to at least 10°DH before the treatment begins.

Method C₁₄

Combination treatment for *Cryptocaryon*
Stock solution: 1 g copper sulfate + 2 g methylene blue + 0.25 g citric acid per 1 liter distilled water.
Carry out the treatment in a separate container. Lower animals do not tolerate the treatment.
Dosage: 12.5 ml stock solutions to 10 liters water. Half the dosage on days four and eight. It is better to keep the copper level between 0.15 and 0.2 mg/Liter. During treatment, filter over cotton or clean foam filter material.

Method C₁₅

Combination treatment for *Cryptocaryon* (according to G.C. Blasiola, *Aquarien Magazine,* 1/81, page 14, Stuttgart, Germany)
Treatment involves two steps. First, the fish are bathed in a short bath (one hour) containing 4 mg copper sulfate + 2.2 ml formalin (37%) to 10 liters seawater in a separate container. Then they are transferred to a long bath containing 20 mg copper per 100 liters sea water. The treatment must last ten days. The short bath can be repeated at a 48-hour intervals.

Method C₁₆

Malachite green oxalate
Use: Ich, other skin protozoans, skin cloudiness or turbidity, and skin fungus.
Spectrum of action: *Ichthyophthirius* spp., *Trichodina* spp., *Chilodonella* spp., *Saprolegnia* spp.

The solution is stable only as long as it is kept cool and away from light. Do not keep malachite green with edibles in the refrigerator because it is highly toxic and carcinogenic. Pet shops stock malachite green preparations, and only when these do not work should the pure substance ever be used.

Dosage A: 6 ml of stock solution to 100 liters of aquarium water. Give half the dosage on days three, six, and nine. After 12 days, change a third of the water. Any water changes needed during treatment must be redosed at the initial strength.

Aeration should be provided during treatment. Malachite green is an intense pigment, and stains can be removed only with difficulty. As a rule, even sensitive fish tolerate this dosage. In water with a heavy organic burden, or in the presence of an active biological filter, the dosage may have to be increased. However, do not exceed a dosage of 15 ml stock solution to 100 liters of aquarium water. If the bath is prepared in a quarantine tank with very pure water and without an already broken-in filter, sensitive fish may not tolerate Dosage A under some circumstances. That is because malachite green is broken down slower in hygienic tanks than it is in tanks with bottom matter and filter. In such tanks the dosage is 4 ml stock solution to 100 liters of aquarium water and then followed up with 2 ml on days four, eight, and 12.

Dosage B: According to G. Blasiola *(Aquarien Magazin,* 9/83, page 477, Stuttgart, Germany), 13-15 mg/100 liters of sea water is effective against *Brooklynella* spp. Treatment is given in a separate tank with filtration over cotton and good aeration for three to four days. It is possible that the above dosage in freshly prepared sea water will not be tolerated.

Method C$_{17}$
Methylene blue
Use: Clouded or turbid skin and mild fungus infections. Prophylaxis against fungal attack on eggs and post-travel stress. Blood diseases (sleeping sickness of fish).

Spectrum of action: *Costia* spp., *Chilodonella* spp., *Trichodina* spp., *Saprolegnia* spp., *Cryptobia* spp., *Trypanosoma* spp.

Methylene blue in a long bath is well liked both as a prophylactic measure and a treatment for disease. It can be administered in the aquarium, though not over activated charcoal, but over freshly washed cotton or foam filter material.

Stock solution: 1 g methylene blue to a liter of water.

Dosage A: 1 ml stock solution to 1 liter water (normal dosage). This dosage can be admininistered in an already set up aquarium. After five days filter over activated charcoal to remove the residual medication.

Dosage B: 3 ml stock solution to 1 liter water (reinforced dosage).

Treatment at this concentration is carried out for five days in a separate container.

Dosage C: Ectoparasites are controlled with a short bath of 200 ml stock solution to 10 liters water for 30 minutes. **Caution:** *Sensitive fish will not tolerate it.*

Dosage D: For prophylaxis against infections after travel, 50 ml of stock solution are added to 100 liters of water in the quarantine tank.

Dosage E: For prophylaxis against fungus attack on eggs, 30 ml of stock solution are added to 100 liters of water in the breeding tank.

Method C$_{18}$
Metriforate, Masoten, Neguvon 100%, trichlorphon
Use: Skin and gill ectoparasites.

Spectrum of action: *Trichodina* spp., *Argulus* spp., *Ergasilus* spp., *Lernaea* spp., *Dactylogyrus* spp., *Gyrodactylus* spp.

Masoten is very toxic and acts vigorously on parasitic crustaceans and skin and gill worms. It is significantly more effective as a long bath than it is as a short one. At higher concentrations, from 28°C up it is toxic to many species of fish. Large species tolerate it better than do smaller ones. Characins and catfish are particularly sensitive. It has been repeatedly claimed Masoten makes fish infertile. That is wrong. Healthy progeny have repeatedly been bred from fish that were treated with high doses of Masoten (3 mg/L for three days).

Treatment can be carried out in the aquarium. Only very dry powder (which looks slightly bluish) can be used; if it forms clumps, then it is unusable. Masoten stored in apparently tightly sealed screw-top jars loses its effect over several months and becomes more toxic. Tests have shown that this loss of effectiveness is associated with the ability to absorb atmospheric humidity. The greater the moisture absorbed, the less the effect on gill worms and the greater the toxicity to fish. Newly purchased Masoten is significantly tolerated better by all fish than is the stored product. This aging process can be delayed by immediately repacking freshly purchased Masoten into tightly closing vials and then storing these, along with a desiccant, in larger glass containers such as jars, or the vials can be sealed in plastic bags. Blue silica gel is an ideal desiccant, the blue granules losing their color when maximum moisture has been absorbed. The gel can be regenerated by spreading it on a tin baking sheet and heating for about 15 minutes at 105° to 110°C. When the moisture is driven off, it turns blue again. This can be done for years.

The quantities given here refer to newly purchased Masoten (assuming, of course, the source's stock is stored properly). For Neguvon, multiply the quantities given by a factor of 0.8.

Stock Solution: 1 g Masoten to 1 liter water.

The solution must be used immediately because it is not stable. Residues must not be dumped into the sewage line before they are neutralized by raising the pH above 12 with sodium hydroxide for two hours.

Dosage A: 100 ml stock solution to 100 liters aquarium water. This concentration is tolerated well by almost all fish if the temperature is at 25°C and the pH between 6 and 7. The treatment lasts three days, after which at least 50% of the water is changed. The residual medication is filtered out over activated charcoal.

Dosage B: 1 g Masoten to 10 liters water as a short bath at 25°C, pH 6 to 7, for one hour in a separate container.

The method with Dosage A (above) is better for controlling livebearing gill and skin worms. With egg-laying *Dactylogyrus* species treatment is not so simple because the eggs can tolerate high levels of Masoten (Chapter 7.2.1.2). With the treatment recommendations described here, a whole population of fish can be freed of gill worms, a method particularly suited to breeding tanks that are free of bottom landscaping and decorations.

Dosage C: The fish are treated according to Dosage A for three days in their aquarium. Then all are caught and transferred to a parasite-free tanks. The original tank can then be washed out, the tubing and filter rinsed, the filter material washed and boiled for half an hour or disinfected with a formalin solution. Then the aquarium is left at least three days to dry out. On day eight following the start of treatment, Dosage A is begun in the second tank and continued for three days. Meanwhile, the first aquarium is refilled with water and the filtration system started up. Following the bath in the second tank, the fish can be returned to their own tank on day 11. The filter needs a run-in time of at least three to six weeks. The temperature cannot go above 25°C throughout the whole treatment process. Only at this temperature is there any guarantee that the larvae that hatched following the first treatment have not developed into sexually mature worms by the start of the second course of treatment.

This method does not effect a permanent cure because some of the *Dactylogyrus* eggs survive weeks or even months at the bottom of the aquarium before they develop further. In this case, method C_6 (flubendazol) is significantly simpler and easier on the fish, and it provides the absolute assurance that no more gill worms will appear after just one treatment.

In general, Masoten should not be used without careful consideration; many fatalities have indicated that handling this drug is not without its problems. Outdated and highly toxic stocks are often used. Its toxicity varies according to fish species and water characteristics; it increases as treatment duration lengthens. High doses are usually tolerated well during the first 24 hours. In no case should fish be put into used solutions or into solutions that are several hours old! Masoten must be administered fresh each time. The residual stock solution must be immediately neutralized with sodium hydroxide and discarded.

Method C_{19}
Metronidazole, flagyl (250 mg)
Use: Flagellate infections in the intestine and organs.

Spectrum of action: *Hexamita* spp., *Spironucleus* spp., *Trichomonas* spp.; *Protoopalina* spp., it does not help against worms.

Flagyl is used as a long bath in the already setup aquarium. The tablets are crushed and first dissolved in lukewarm water, then distributed over the surface of the water in the aquarium. The temperature can be raised to 30-33°C to support the treatment.

Dosage: 250 mg (one tablet) to 50 liters of aquarium water. After three days, change one-third of the water and gradually lower the temperature. Filter over activated charcoal to remove the drug from the water. Sensitive plants may be affected for a while.

Dosage in feed: Crush a 250 mg tablet of flagyl into powder and, at 50°C, mix it into the feed prepared by method B_5. Administer it morning and evening for six days.

Method C$_{20}$
MS-222 (Tricaine), amino-benzoic acid ethyl ester methansulfonate

MS-222 is one of the best proven fish anesthetics. It also acts on many lower animals and is used in microscopy to tranquilize microorganisms. Its effect on fish attenuates with increasing water hardness.

Dosage A: (to tranquilize fish for travel): 10 mg per liter of water.

Dosage B: (to anesthetize fish when taking smears): From 50 to 130 mg per liter of water, depending upon size of fish (Reichenbach-Klinke, 1980). Transfer the fish to fresh water after 15 minutes at the very latest and let it recuperate there for another 15 minutes.

Dosage C: (to sacrifice fish): 1 g to 1 liter of water kills in 10 minutes.

Method C$_{21}$
Nitrofurantoin (gelatin capsules each containing 100 mg active ingredient)

Use: Turbid (or cloudy fins) and fin rot (bath), external bacterial infections, prevent spread of abdominal dropsy, bacterial infection of kidney, vibriosis.

Spectrum of action: Some Gram-positive bacteria, *Pseudomonas* spp., *Aeromonas* spp., *Vibrio* spp.

If bacterially infected fish are transferred out of the aquarium and into a quarantine tank, then the remaining fish can be treated prophylactically with nitrofurantoin. This medication can be administered in the aquarium if the filter material is first cleaned off and the bottom mulm aspirated out of the tank. Activated charcoal must be removed from the filter.

Dosage: Add the content of one nitrofurantoin capsule to 30-40 liters of aquarium water. The capsule halves can be easily pulled apart to reach the ingredients, which are dissolved in a beaker of warm water and poured along with any undissolved residue into the aquarium being treated. The long bath lasts 15 days. Afterward, change a large portion of the water and filter it over charcoal.

Dosage in feed: Add 300 mg pulverized nitrofurantoin (the contents of three capsule) to 200 g of the feed made by method B$_5$ and administer morning and evening for nine days.

Method C$_{22}$
Furazolidone (1 g cachet or envelope containing 300 mg active ingredient and 700 mg glucose)

This drug is cheap but can only be administered in feed. The active ingredient is available only in 500 g packages, thus is relatively expensive. Pure furazolidone can be given alone, without other substances, as a short bath.

Use: *Pseudomonas* spp., *Aeromonas* spp., *Vibrio* spp., *Trichomonas* spp., and many *coccidia.*

Dosage in feed: Add, at 50-55°C, 300 mg furazolidone to 100 g of feed made according to method B$_5$ and feed morning and evening for six days.

Dosage for long bath: 500 mg pure furazolidone to 100 liters water in separate tank. Do not filter over charcoal. Change 40% to 50% of the water after three days. Residual medication can be removed from the water by filtration over activated charcoal.

Method C$_{23}$
Nystatin ointment

The ointment base consists of liquid polyethylene and liquid parafin, and it adheres particularly well to skin and mucosa.

Use: Fungal infections of skin, and prophylaxis for wounds.

Spectrum of action: Fungi.

Lift the fish out of the water, carefully use blotting or filter paper to dry off the affected area, and then apply Nystatin ointment.

Duration of treatment: One to two times daily until the fungal hyphae disappear, the wound closes, or new skin forms.

Method C$_{24}$
Piperazine citrate

Use: Intestinal worms.

Spectrum of action: Thorny-headed worms, tapeworms, trematodes.

Piperazine citrate must be administered with feed so that it can act directly in the gut. Since it is heat-stable, it can be mixed into the hot feed (prepared by method B$_5$) at 80°C.

Dosage: Mix 600 mg piperazine citrate into 100/g feed (made by method B$_5$ and feed once morning and evening on days one and eight.

Method C$_{25}$
Sulfonamides, sulfathiazole

Sulfonamides are available from several manufacturers and under various trade names.

Use: Internal bacterial infections.

Spectrum of action: Actinomycetes, cocci, and many Gram-positive and a few Gram-negative bacteria, *Pseudomonas* spp., flexibacteria, corynebacteria.

Since sulfonamides pass well from the gut to the blood, mixing it into the feed is its most effective application. It is the drug of choice particularly in infections of the internal organs caused by the above organisms.

Dosage: Mix 300 mg sulfathiazole into 100 g of the feed prepared by method B$_5$. The temperature should be 60°C. Administer the feed morning and evening for three days.

The poor solubility of the drug makes its use difficult in a long bath. It is given in a separate container. First dissolve the weighed amount of medication in warm (up to 60°C) water in a closed vessel by agitating it for a minute. **Caution:** Since the enclosed air sharply expands in the closed vessel, it can explode! After the first shake, let the excess air escape. After shaking, distribute it over the surface of the water in the treatment tank, which should not contain a filter, otherwise it would filter out the finely suspended sulfa drug. To prevent it from settling out on the bottom, the water has to be kept vigorously circulating with a power head.

Method C$_{26}$
Trimethoprim

Use: Bacterial and coccal infections of internal organs and blood.

Spectrum of action: Staphylococci, hemolytic streptococci, pneumococci, *Escherichia coli,* enterococci, *Proteus, Hemophilus influenzae, Salmonella, Shigella.*

Combining trimetoprim with a sulfonamide offers a significant improvement in efficacy. There are ready-made combinations available of trimethoprim and sulfamethoxazole in optimal proportions. Since pathogens develop resistance very rapidly, the medication should be used only once every six months.

Commercially available preparations include: Drylin, Eusaprim, Borgal solution (7.5%), and Cotrimstada-forte. Drylin and Eusaprim are older preparations with low concentrations of active ingredient. Today (in Europe) the most commonly used preparations are Borgal and Cotrimstada-forte.

Dosage: 1 table Cotrimstada-forte to 80 liters aquarium water for three to five days. The filter cannot contain any charcoal; the filter floss has to be washed out thoroughly before administration of the drug.

15 ml Borgal solution to 100 liters water.

For injection, calculate 2 ml Borgal solution (7.5%) per 200 g body weight. A second injection can be given if necessary after 48 hours. The injection is given intraperitoneally.

Only veterinarians and other experts should immunize or vaccinate fish.

Method C$_{27}$
Vitamin preparations

Commercially available preparations for aquarists bind the vitamins to water-insoluble powder or oil to prevent their volatilization and loss and to facilitate their adherence to the feed particles until the fish ingests them. It is important that they also include calcium and phosphorus to cure hole-in-the-head disease once the cause is removed (Chapter 9.3). Many other substances and trace elements have a positive influence on the health and color of fish. Preparations that contain vitamins dissolved in water (aqueous solutions) are not very effective since they become dispersed in the aquarium water and are quickly decomposed.

Mix 500 mg vitamin powder into 100 g feed, which should not be fed to healthy fish more than twice a week. It can be given to sick fish, though, four to five times a week. Once these fish recover, the dosage is reduced to the normal one.

Excessive feeding of vitamins to fish causes signs and symptoms of disease (Chapter 9.3).

When using Osspulvit - N or Calcipot in feed prepared according to methods B$_4$ and B$_5$, any missing vitamins or minerals must be replaced by other preparations. The use of pulverized VMP tablets (Pfizer) is a possibility.

Method C$_{28}$
Volon-A adhesive ointment

This ointment possesses outstanding characteristics of adherence to skin and mucosa, which must be dried off first (as described in method C$_{23}$). It is used for wounds and skin infections by applying it as a layer of ointment over the affected areas. The active ingredient is anti-inflammatory, which means that even extensive skin wounds can be covered with it. If necessary, powdered antibiotics, sulfonamides, or antimycotic (antifungal) agents can be mixed into the ointment.

Dosage: Work the powdered active ingredient (5% by volume) into the ointment (95%).

Method C$_{29}$
Hydrogen peroxide (3%)

In addition to disinfection, hydrogen peroxide can also be used to rapidly increase oxygen in aquarium water. It decomposes into water by liberating pure oxygen.

Add 25 ml of 3% hydrogen peroxide to 100 liters of aquarium water (Krause, 1985). In no case can the dosage be given a second time. Overdosage with oxygen would corrode the gills and skin of the fish, resulting in their death. If the fish do not breathe easier within several minutes following dosage, then the lack of oxygen has another cause (for example, gill parasites)

Method D$_1$
Potassium permanganate

Potassium permanganate is used to disinfect aquariums and utensils that cannot be boiled (tubing, thermometers, etc.). Fill the aquarium up to the brim with water and put in it all the items to be disinfected. Then add enough potassium permanganate until the violet color of the water is so intense that you cannot see through the tank anymore. Let the external filter run without any filter medium so the violet solution rinses all parts of it. After three days empty the tank and rinse it with clean water until all the color is washed away.

Method D$_2$
Table salt

Salt can be used for disinfection. Dissolve 350 g salt in 1 liter of water. Disinfection of an aquarium in this way would be expensive and inconvenient, but the method is ideal to sterilize nets and other small utensils.

Prepare a bucket containing a salt solution at this concentration and leave the nets standing in it. A net should be in it 24 hours before being reused. Since the salt solution never goes bad or gets weaker, a bucketful lasts a long time. Use tap water to replace water from the bucket as it evaporates. If you color it slightly with a little methylene blue, it will not be confused with other buckets of solutions.

Empty aquariums can be scrubbed out with a slurry of salt and salt solution. Let the slurry dry on the glas panes of the tank and repeat the whole operation another five times over the next few days.

Method D$_3$
Hydrogen peroxide (30%)

Caution: Hydrogen peroxide at 30% concentration is highly corrosive. Do not let this product come into contact with skin or clothing.

Hydrogen peroxide can be decomposed into oxygen and ordinary water by light, thus it is stored in brown or amber bottles. To disinfect an empty aquarium, add 50 ml of 30% hydrogen peroxide to 100 liters of water. Landscaping articles and utensils can go into the solution. Gravel is best disinfected by baking it at 150°C for two hours (not counting warm-up time), otherwise the hydrogen peroxide will be exhausted too quickly. Let the filter operate, but without any contents (see D$_1$). Let the solution stand in the tank for three days, with the lamp turned on during this time. Then empty the tank and rinse it out with tap water. The advantage of this method is that it does not leave any residual matter that would have to be meticulously cleaned out later.

Method D$_4$
Alum

Disinfection of plants is the major use of alum in aquariums. At pet shops, water plants that are not kept in separate plant tanks but in tanks along with fish could transmit pathogens and their various resting stages to your aquarium at home. Because these plants do not do well in quarantine tanks, you have to disinfect them before replanting them in the aquarium. Dissolve a heaped teaspoon of alum in a liter of water and soak the plants in it for five minutes. Then rinse them off thoroughly with fresh water before planting in the aquarium.

Method D$_5$
Isopropanol, isopropyl alcohol
Many aquarists may feel the need to disinfect their hands in addition to washing them after autopsy of a fish. That is, as a rule, not necessary since fish diseases generally are not transmitted to man. Tuberculosis, however, is an exception.

Commercially available 100% isopropanol is diluted to 70% (U.S. drugstores often carry several strengths, one of which is 70%). To dilute, measure off 70 ml of the 100% isopropanol in a graduated cylinder, then simply add enough water to bring it up to the 100 ml mark. Then, after washing them with soap and water, wet your hands with this alcohol and let them dry in the air. This 70% working solution is also good for soaking small utensils and tubing to disinfect them.

If you fill a spray bottle (such as used for spraying a water mist on plants) with 70% isopropanol, you can disinfect empty tanks and other large objects with it. Spray all surfaces, particularly the hard-to-reach-inside corners, thoroughly and evenly, then let them dry. Repeat the spraying in a few hours. The alcohol evaporates without leaving any residue, so the aquarium can be filled up again after the alcohol dries.

Method D$_6$
Formalin
Add 30 ml of the normally available 35-40% formalin to a 10-liter bucket (that can be closed with a cover) and fill with water to capacity. To avoid confusion, color the solution with methylene blue. Nets and other small objects can be dipped into this solution. A two-hour bath disinfects with absolute certainty.

This method is not without its risks in an enclosed area, since formalin (actually formaldehyde) fumes in the air can irritate the respiratory passages. Working with formalin solutions can irritate the skin. In addition, remember that formalin is carcinogenic.

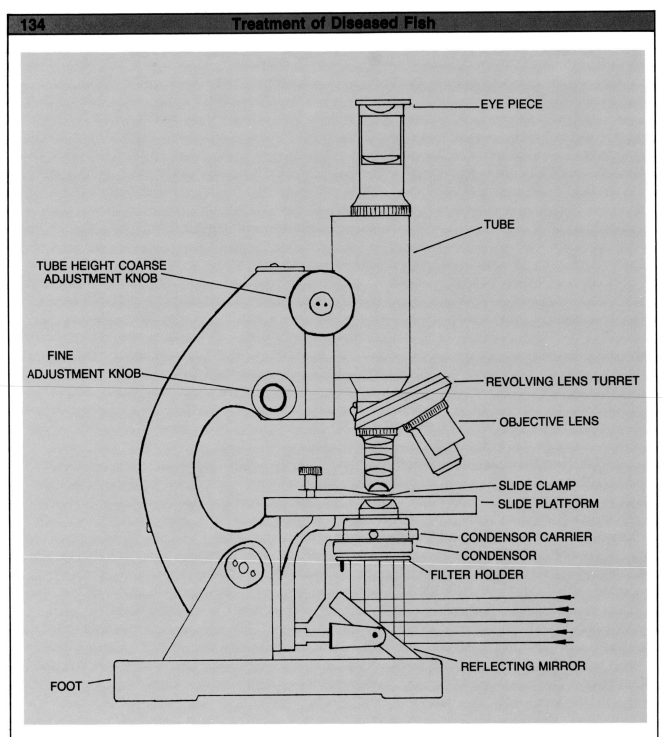

EYE PIECE

TUBE

TUBE HEIGHT COARSE
ADJUSTMENT KNOB

FINE
ADJUSTMENT KNOB

REVOLVING LENS TURRET

OBJECTIVE LENS

SLIDE CLAMP
SLIDE PLATFORM

CONDENSOR CARRIER
CONDENSOR
FILTER HOLDER

REFLECTING MIRROR

FOOT

108. An economical student microscope.

Chapter 11

MICROSCOPY IN THE DIAGNOSIS OF FISH DISEASES

11.1. The Microscope

The most important tool for diagnosing fish diseases is the microscope (Photograph No. 108). It is indispensable for examining smears, parasites, and organ specimens. A child's microscope is inexpensive, yet of no use in this work. Most do not have standard parts, and the optical systems are inadequate. Children and young students lose their interest quickly, or, if against all expectations this does not happen, they eventually come into possession of a first-rate microscope. A good microscope's high price can easily scare you, but keep in mind that an instrument like that, with proper care, does not wear out, so the investment is not too high. A good microscope is an acquisition for life.

All suppliers of good microscopes make it possible to begin with a basic outfit and then, over time as means allow, expanding and improving. This chapter does not have the scope to develop an introduction to microscopic technique. The beginner is advised to carefully study the instructions and other literature that come with a newly purchased microscope. Technical literature for beginners as well as for advanced microscopists abounds.

When buying a microscope, make sure that all connections are standard. If the tube length is 160 mm, the products of many manufacturers can be combined with it. Good lens are engraved with the length of the matching tube.

In the beginning, objective lenses of 10X, 20X, and 40X magnification are sufficient. To match those are three oculars or eyepiece lenses, with 5X, 10X, and 15X magnification. The maximum magnification with these lenses is 600X (i.e., 40 x 15 = 600X), adequate for studying fish parasites. As you get deeper into microscopy, you can obtain lenses with up to 100X magnification (making 100 x 15 = 1500X magnification possible).

Microscope stands are built two different ways. In one, the tube is raised or lowered to focus; in the other, the stage rises or falls. The stand with the fixed tube and movable stage is sturdier.

Besides normal brightfield illumination, other illumination methods are available. The best known are the darkfield and phase contrast methods. While only an experienced practitioner with knowledge of instrumentation can whip up a phase contrast setup at home, a darkfield arrangement for going up to 400X is easy to put together. To do that, cut circular pieces of various diameters from black cardboard. The diameter of the central aperture for high magnification lenses is larger than for those with weak magnification. The apertures are set consecutively in the middle of a glass disc or clear film that fits in the filter holder. A circular field of varying width is created, depending upon how much the condenser aperture opens (Photograph No. 109). You test the various apertures for each lens until one produces a uniformly intense black field in which the object shines brightly. Even the smaller bacteria can be seen well at 400X magnification. The impressive effect occurs when the circular light from the condenser forms a concave sphere, the apex of which lies in the object's field, though upside down. It spreads above so that the direct light is directed past the object. The field of vision is dark while the object diverts the incident light into the lens and thus seems bright. All darkfield photographs in this book were made with such homemade apertures.

11.2. Measurement at the Microscopic Level

The power of a lens is often cited in descriptions, drawings, and photographs. This is not given as microscopic magnification,

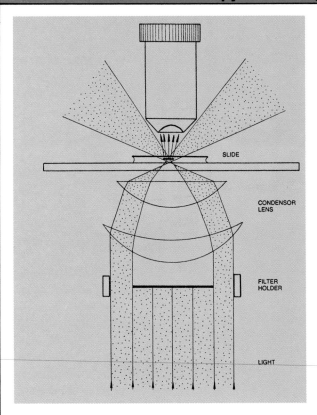

109. Dark field setup.

the ocular micrometer, then the calculation is 0.93 mm: 59 divisions = 0.01576 mm = 15.76 microns per each division.

From now on, only the ocular micrometer is needed, and you know that one division of its scale = 15.76 microns. So, for example, a worm 86 divisions long is 1355 microns or 1.35 mm.

For readers who do not have ocular micrometers, here is a list of approximate micron values for one division when working with most common lenses, with a 10X measuring ocular etched with a 10-mm scale divided into 100 parts:

Lens	Micron
2.5X	83.2
4X	23.8
5X	20
6.3X	15.8
10X	9.8
16X	6.3
20X	5.1
25X	3.8
40X	2.44
63X	1.68
100X	1

These values vary slightly according to the manufacturer of the lenses. The tube magnification has to be 1X for this to work.

110. Micrometer and graduated ocular with measuring scale.

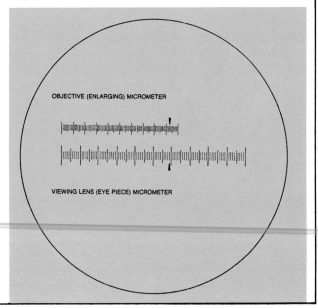

OBJECTIVE (ENLARGING) MICROMETER

VIEWING LENS (EYE PIECE) MICROMETER

as specimen size in microns, thus obviating any errors in photographs and drawing that may be photographically enlarged later. The viewer can calculate the magnification himself by measuring the size of the image and dividing it by the stated size of the object. To measure an object's size, one uses an ocular micrometer or eyepiece calibrated with a 10-mm scale divided into 100 parts. To match the lens to this scale, a specimen micrometer is needed, but only once, so it can be borrowed from a friend. The specimen micrometer is a stage upon which a 1-mm scale (with 100 divisions) is engraved. For every lens, the value for one part of the ocular micrometer must be calculated. Lay the specimen micrometer on the stage in such a way that the beginnings of both scales coincide (Photograph No. 110). Then look for a spot where two lines exactly coincide. The further toward the end of the scale that this happens, the more accurate the result. If, for example, 93 divisions of the specimen micrometer coincide with 59 divisions of

11.3. Glassware

In addition to the microscope and the instruments mentioned in Chapter 3.1, a few more items are needed:

1. Glass slides and cover glasses or cover slips are the first items to mention. The slides are 76 x 26 mm glass strips. Cover slips are 0.17 mm thick and usually 18 x 22 mm square, or round.
2. Glass pipettes can be drawn from glass tubing that has been softened in the flame of a Bunsen or other burner. The appropriate length is scratched off, slightly filed through with a glass file, and then snapped off. Little suction balls or caps are placed on the ends of the pipettes.
3. Graduated pipettes can measure small volumes of liquid up to 0.1 ml.
4. A 100-ml graduated cylinder measures large quantities of liquids.
5. Two to three small glass dishes (watch-glasses, evaporating dishes, or Petri dishes) are needed for observation of small specimens with a magnifying glass.
6. Five shallow preparation or dissecting containers of glass with tightly fitting tops are needed for staining, etc. Small Petri dishes (60 mm in diameter) with covers are also suitable.

11.4. Live Specimens

The most expensive instrument is worthless if you cannot use it properly. To practice microscopy or even to familiarize yourself with it, you have to first prepare a simple specimen. To do that, put a drop of water on a microscope slide and add a few algal filaments to it. Then cover with a cover slip, which takes some practice to do without capturing any air bubbles underneath. Hold the cover slip between thumb and forefinger or with forceps at a 45° angle to the glass slide so that the specimen drop is in the angle, then draw it slowly backwards until it contacts the drop of water. The water will now spread under the cover glass along the edge making contact. Now slowly and uniformly lower the other edge of the cover slip so that the drop of water forces out the air without leaving any bubbles underneath. In a well-made preparation, the space between cover slip and slide must not be thicker than the cover slip itself.

If a thicker specimen is to be mounted, the space under the cover slip must be filled with water. Mounts that are too thick do not let light through too well at higher powers and only the uppermost layer can be focused sharply. That is because the depth of the sharply focused level becomes shallower as the power of magnification increases. This depth of field or sharpness plane can be represented by a more or less thin layer that lies parallel to the cover slip and runs through the specimen; everything that is sharp to the viewer is in this plane. At first, it takes some practice to develop a feel for the size of the water drop that contains the specimen.

Algal filaments make good practice specimens because you can make very thin mounts from them. Excess water can be blotted away by holding filter paper or a blotter at the edge of the cover slip. Take care not to let very small specimens get sucked out along with the excess water (due to capillary action). The same procedure applies when making other fresh mounts and smears.

Now the mount can be placed on the microscope stage. The manufacturer's instructions explain how to obtain the best lighting. Take care to avoid any contact of the objectives (the rotating lenses) with the fingers or with the mount, since these lenses may become scratched or greasy. For that reason, coarse focusing never proceeds toward the slide mount, but always away from it. Bring your eye down to see horizontally across the stage as you turn the objective down to the slide so that it almost touches the slide. Then look into the ocular and turn the coarse focusing wheel so that the objectives rise until the object just begins to appear as an out-of-focus image. Now turn the fine focus knob to focus sharply.

When working with dead fish, it is a good idea to prepare beforehand several slides with water drops into which to transfer specimens you are going to dissect out of the fish. The cover slips, too, should be clean, dry, and free of oily or greasy spots (such as fingerprints).

Pick up slides and cover slips only by the edges, never in the middle, to avoid finger oils.

Many slides and cover slips are cleaned before packaging, but that is not clean enough for good mounts. Lay the slides and cover slips in a small vessel of alcohol before they are needed, when you can lift them out with forceps and dry them off with an absorbent cloth. If that is too inconvenient, fill another vessel (which can be tightly closed) with chloroform, then take the slide and cover slip from the alcohol, dip them into the chloroform, wave them with the forceps for a few seconds in the air, and both slide and cover slip, now free of oils and clean, will dry quickly.

Used slides and cover slips are cleaned for reuse only when they are not too soiled, which occurs only when you used them for specimens prepared with water. If specimens are fixed and stained, however, it really takes too much time and effort to attempt to clean off the slides. The beginner has a hard time trying to clean cover slips, most of which break when being wiped.

Whoever wants to work with fish diseases must not be satisfied merely to examine a sick fish from time to time. A serious study of microorganisms and aquatic biology is generally required to be able to differentiate harmless from parasitic organisms and to recognize the cause of disease. This learning process is definitely not boring, and whoever has once observed the microorganisms in a drop of water with a good microscope will certainly always enjoy microscopy. The bottom matter and filter of an aquarium are true treasure troves once you have learned to recognize the harmless protozoa, worms, and arthropods hidden there. These organisms can be identified with the help of various guides and books available in libraries and bookshops. Photographs Nos. 111 to 115 show some of the harmless inhabitants of the aquarium.

11.5. Teased Fragment and Squash Mounts

To prepare organs for microscopic examinations, small bits the size of pinheads are used to make thin transparent mounts that can be sharply focused. Place a bit in a drop of physiological saline (0.64%) on a glass slide and tease it with two sharp needles (dissecting needles) into the smallest particles or shreds

you can make. If the specimen is still too thick to allow placement of the cover slip, a clean, blunt object can be pressed down on the cover slip just above the largest fragment (being careful not to crack the cover slip). Now place the mount on the microscope stage and start with the lowest power to study the specimen. Chapter 3 describes when specimens should be teased into fragments and when they should be squashed whole under glass.

Squash mounts require some force. Place the bit of organ tissue between two glass slides, without any water, and press together (without sliding or shearing) until the tissue bit is spread out extremely thin. Then add some water to this thinned-out specimen and lay a cover slip over it.

11.6. Isolation of Pathogens

If one or more parasites are found in a fresh specimen, they are often transferred to a new mount. There are several reasons for this. The microscopist may want to get a better look at the parasite, or perhaps be able to photograph it alone so it stands out clearly. Also, if permanent mounts are going to be prepared, the parasite must be taken out of the fresh mount and treated further. To do this, lay the glass slide on a glass plate or pane that can be lighted from underneath. For a light source,

111. *Stentor* occur in every aquarium. They live on soil and plants. Size: 0.1 to 2mm.

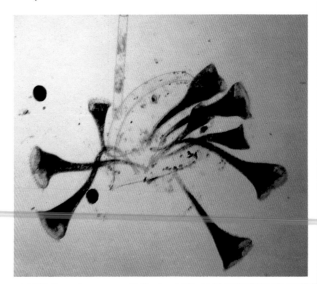

you can use a bulb (such as from a desk lamp) and reflect the light with a mirror up through the glass and the specimen lying on it (Photograph No. 116). The light can be softened by using a sheet of tracing paper in front of the mirror as a diffuser. Now use a strong hand lens or loupe to look down on the specimen to see the parasite(s). A magnifier on a stand is a practical way to have both hands free. Raise the cover slip carefully with pointed forceps. If the specimen sticks to it, loosen it with a dissecting needle. It is easier, however, to transfer the specimen from the slide into a small circular dish (watchglass, Petri dish) filled with two to three milliliters with physiological saline (see chapter 10, method C$_{12}$).

Now use two dissecting needles to free the parasite from the surrounding tissue. Tease apart intestinal fragments or cut them lengthwise. Many parasites can last several hours in

112. *Stylaria* worms wriggle along under the surface of the water. They measure 1mm at most in thickness, but up to 4cm in length. The photograph shows the head.

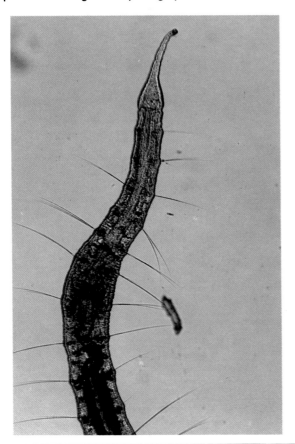

this solution, so there is no great rush in completing the procedures. Using a finely drawn-out pipette, you can suck up the parasites individully and transfer them to a small drop of physiological saline on clean slides. After covering with a cover slip, examine at 100 to 300X. Larger parasites can easily be crushed under the cover slip, so it is advisable to prevent too close a contact by using spacers to prevent the cover slip from pressing down too closely. Affix tiny modeling clay or wax pellets to the corners of the cover slip so as to form little feet turned inward toward the specimen as the slip is placed on the slide, then tap gently with a dissecting needle on the cover slip until it settles down low enough to clamp the specimen in place. If any water is needed, put it in at the edge. Now the living specimen can be observed without rushing. Extremely small parasites such as flagellates in the blood and intestine are not visible under a loupe or handlens. For these, place the uncovered mount on the microscope stage again and search under a low power for a spot containing many flagellates. Then suck up the fluid containing these with a very finely drawn pipette. Transfer that to a waiting slide that you have arleady provided with a tiny drop of physiological slaine. This new mount will be very thin, thus allowing examination under very high power.

It is sometimes necessary to keep fresh mounts for several days so we can study the course of the pathogen's development. Keep it in a humid room to prevent the mount's water from evaporating. In a tightly closing glass jar or dish containing water to a height of 2 centimeters, lay the slide on a pedestal or stand that just rises above the level of the water. Only the underside of the slide has to be wiped off before it is placed under the microscope for examination.

11.7. Preparation of Specimens in General

In many cases it becomes necessary to keep parasites for lengthy periods of time, perhaps as a reference slide against which to compare new specimens later, or perhaps to take to an expert for identification. The problem is to preserve these microorganisms that long. That is achieved either by preserving them in solvent mixtures or by preparing permanent mounts of them. They also can be stained while they are being worked up.

Several steps are necessary to make permanent mounts. The first one is fixing or fixation. The specimen is put into a fixative or fixing solution that kills the cells but leaves the tissues in a life-like condition. They will not decompose and the whole organism keeps its shape. Fixation also prepares the specimen for further processing. It allows the protein to coagulate so that the cell membranes become transparent and dyes can penetrate the cells.

Good fixation requires that the fixative be able to penetrate quickly. For that reason, the specimen should not be thicker than 1 centimeter at any spot. The quantity of fluid amounts to 50 to 100 times the volume of the specimen. The fixative has to act a certain amount of time and can only be used once. Sometimes the fixative solution must be rinsed off the specimen after fixation, which is done by soaking the specimen in distilled water or in alcohol for a certain time. In the following guidelines for preparing mounts, the steps and times for soaking the specimens in the solutions are given. With these guidelines, the beginner can prepare usable slides that give him the option of sending them for expert diagnosis.

Since fixation must be done fast, larger specimens are always soaked in a prepared fixative bath. They are then taken out with finely pointed forceps or pipetted up with a finely drawn out pipette. Keep as much water out of the fixative as possible. Nematodes can be easily caught and transferred with a dissecting needle.

The specimens to be fixed contain a great deal of water that must be removed because it would not mix with the imbedding material (usually plastics). Various strengths of alcohol are needed to dehydrate the specimen. Depending upon which fixative is used, start with 20 to 40% alcohol, increasing the concentration stepwise by 10 to 15% each time until the specimen reaches pure alcohol. You can prepare the different concentrations yourself according to the following instructions; keep the

solutions in tightly closed bottles because alcohol absorbs atmospheric moisture, thus diluting itself.

The specimens can be transferred directly into the same strength of alcohol as the strength of the alcohol in the fixative mixture. All steps should be done in a liquid volume that is 50 to 100 times that of the specimen. The individual steps are carried out in small watchglasses or shallow dishes covered with a glass plate.

The specimen can be either transferred from step to step, or else the fixative pipetted off and then replaced with the next concentration, which must be done completely. To prevent sucking up any specimen, observe the tip of the pipette with a loupe (magnifying glass) while pipetting.

In this way the specimens progress through the alcohol series until they reach an alcohol concentration of 70%, in which they can be stored for one to two days. The vessel, of course, must be airtight. Specimens not intended for staining will continue through the remaining steps until they reach the 100% alcohol. For concentrations over 60%, isopropyl alcohol is best because pharmacies stock this in 100% form (at least in some places). Dilute as described earlier into the required concentrations. Pure ethyl alcohol is free of water but only available professionally or with a prescription; even if you purchased it from a wholesale manufacturer, it is too expensive for this work.

From the pure isopropyl alcohol, the specimens are transferred into xylol, which must be changed once. After the indicated length of the bath, prepare one or several carefully cleaned microscope slides by placing one drop of imbedding material in the middle. Now fish the specimens out of the xylol and transfer one to three of them to the drop of balsam (e.g., Entellan), arrange them with the dissecting needle, then seal it over with a clean cover slip, taking care to avoid bubbles. Let the mount dry undisturbed and dust-free for several hours to days.

In thicker mounts, the imbedding balsam may shrivel. In that case, add more imbedding material at the edges of the cover slip several times over the next few days. Then, if the shrinkage stops, use a xylol-soaked cloth to wipe off the excess balsam from the edges of the cover slip and the slide.

Now the mount can be labeled with two adhesive labels cut to fit the empty spaces at the right end and the left end of the slide. The following information must be given:

One end	Other end
Fixative	Origin (if a parasite, give host and organ)
Stain	Name of preparer
Imbedding substance	Date prepared
Latin (binomial) name	

The dry slide can now be numbered and stored horizontally in a slide box. The protocol card that describes the autopsy is given a matching number and then filed away. Thus the slide and protocol are cross-indexed and are always available.

There can be many reasons to stain a slide mount. The simplest reason is that it makes the specimen easier to find under the microscope. Double staining shows the internal organs in one color and the surrounding tissues in another color. The procedure for staining depends upon which fixative was used and the stain. If the fixative contained alcohol, then the specimen can go right into a stain that is dissolved in alcohol.

If, however, a stain is to be used that is dissolved in water, then the specimen has to go backward through the series of alcohol concentrations until it floats in pure distilled water. After staining, the specimen must once again run up through the alcohol series before it passes through xylol and then is placed in the imbedding substance on a slide and sealed with the cover glass.

If the specimen has remained too long in the staining solution and is overstained to the point of becoming opaque, then the excess stain can be dissolved out by means of certain solutions, a process called differentiation. Then the specimen can either be counterstained or dehydrated in the alcohol series, soaked in xylol, and imbedded in plastic.

The times given later for how long to leave specimens in staining solutions and the alcohol series are average values that may be modified according to your experience and the size of the specimens.

If mounts are to be kept longer than a few weeks, then the opening between cover slip and slide must be hermetically sealed. An enamel or shellac is available for sealing. It is painted several times with a small brush around the edges of the coverslip, overlapping in such a way that the cover slip seems to merge right into the slide, leaving no gaps. The mount is then preserved permanently.

The preparation of microorganisms is an intriguing activity for the microscopist, who, as time goes along, will develop a valuable collection of permanent mounts that is always available as a reference for comparison against new specimens. You should practice this technique occasionally with readily available specimens, so that when rare parasites come along you will not spoil them.

11.8. Preparation of Specimens in Detail (E_1—E_{10})

Whoever wants to work up a microscopic collection of parasites from fish and other organisms must always have a basic supply of chemicals and dyes available. The needs include:

1 liter alcohol (household)
1 liter distilled water
1 liter 100% isopropyl alcohol
250 ml 35-40% formalin (formaldehyde)
250 ml xylol
250 ml lactic acid
100 ml glycerin
100 ml 100% acetic acid
100 ml 25% hydrochloric acid (HCl)
100 ml methylene blue (Loeffler)
100 ml alcoholic borax carmine
5-10 g methyl green
Various imbedding substances as commercially available (such as glycerin gelatin, polyvinyl-lactophenol, Canada balsam or Entellan)
Shellac or enamel for sealing the edges around cover slips
Bacterial stains such as carbol fuchsin (Ziehl-Neelsen); carbol gentian violet (Gram) 1:2: 300; and fuchsin solution (Gram)
100 ml graduated cylinder calibrated in 1 ml graduations for measuring out liquids

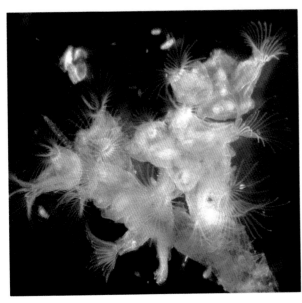

113. *Bryozoa* are colonial polyps. Size of individuals range from 200 to 500u. Colonies can attain several centimeters in size.

First, here is how to set up an alcohol series. Start with spirits that contain 94% ethyl alcohol. To make 30% alcohol, add 30 ml spirits to the graduated cylinder and fill it up with distilled water to the 94 ml mark. To make 60% alcohol, add 60 ml spirits and 34 ml distilled water to make 94 ml liquid. With this procedure, we prepare 30%, 40%, 50%, and 60% alcohol concentrations from spirits. Keep these concentrations in tightly stoppered bottles, each labeled accordingly.

The higher concentrations are made with 100% isopropyl alcohol. Take 70 ml alcohol and fill up to the 100 ml mark with water. With this procedure, we prepare 70%, 80%, 90%, 95%, and 100% concentrations.

Next, here is how to prepare a fixative solution (method E_1) in which worms can be kept for years. To 100 ml spirits (94% alcohol) add 30 ml formalin, 5 ml acetic acid, and 200 ml distilled water, then mix well before storing in an air-tight bottle.

Arthropods such as crustaceans, mites, insects, and insect larvae are fixed in a mixture of 90% spirits and 10% lactic acid (method E_2), in which they can be stored several weeks. Specimens are sent in screw-top vials of these fluids, filled up to keep air out, for expert diagnosis.

11.8.1 Permanent Mounts in Polyvinyl-lactophenol (PVL) (E_3)

The specimen fixed in E_2 (see above) must first be transferred to pure lactic acid before being imbedded in PVL. That can be done stepwise by taking the specimen up through, usually, four stages of lactic acid and alcohol mixtures as follows:

Step 1 = 25% lactic acid + 75% alcohol
Step 2 = 50% lactic acid + 50% alcohol
Step 3 = 80% lactic acid + 20% alcohol
Step 4 = 100% lactic acid.

Since lactic acid decolorizes a specimen, the specimen is kept in the last step until it is translucent, then is transferred to PVL. Delicate arthropods can remain at steps 1 and 2 for several hours. Steps 3 and 4, however, should not last longer than three hours. Check the decolorizing process from time to time with a magnifying glass and interrupt it by imbedding the specimen in the PVL. The specimens

114. *Chaetogaster* spp. become approximately 2mm long.

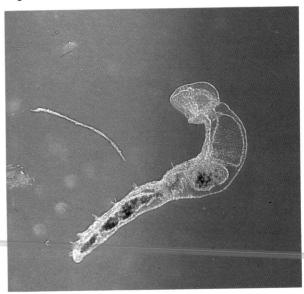

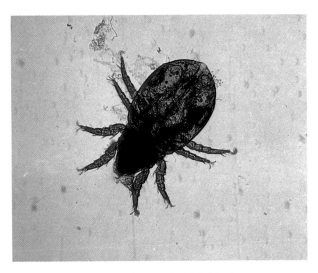

115. Although most mites look frightful, they are competely harmless.

do not have to be too translucent, for they lighten even more over the course of time, even in the completed permanent mount. The mite illustrated in Photograph No. 104 was prepared with this method.

Another possibility for transferring organisms from the fixative mixture to the pure lactic acid is more suited to non-delicate specimens. Fill a small cylindrical glass with some lactic acid and add the specimens along with fixative solution. The fixative solution should not exceed a quarter of the volume of lactic acid. The organisms sink slowly in the lactic acid and can be transferred directly into the PVL.

116. Homemade laboratory bench.

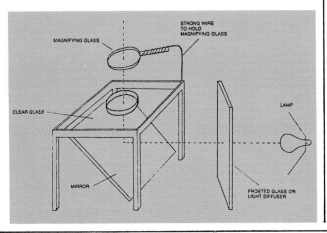

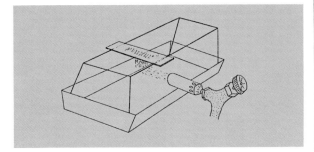

117. Staining rack of stiff wire in a plastic photo developing tray.

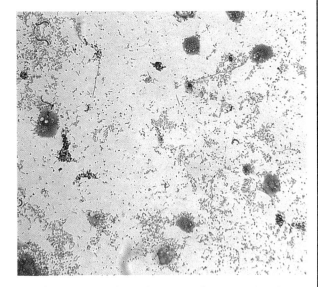

118. Gram-stained fish skin smear. Gram-positive: blue-black. Gram-negative: red. Picture width: 345u.

119. *Mycobacterium* (red with Ziehl-Neelsen stain). Picture length: 120u.

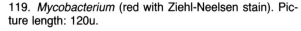
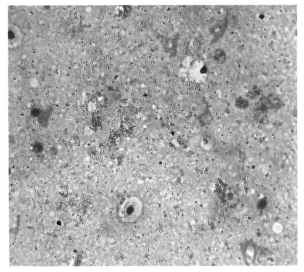

Prepare a large drop of PVL on an clean slide. Transfer the organisms with a dissecting needle from the lactic acid to the PVL. Cover with a cover slip. When preparing larger specimens, use spacers (clay or wax pellets) to keep the cover slip from crushing the specimens. Store the slides horizontally and, if necessary, add more PVL daily under the edges of the coverslip. On the third day, wait until the last PVL added has dried, scratch off the excess imbedding substance with a pointed knife, and seal the cover slip. If you wait any longer, shrinkage can occur. Water fleas and small insects make good practice specimens with which to develop skill at preparing slides.

11.8.2 Permanent Mounts in Canada Balsam or Entellan (E₄)

This method of preparation is well suited to tapeworms and arthropods. Nematodes (roundworms) are somewhat delicate and shrink easily, so they must be handled very carefully if this method is used for them.

The parasites dissected out of the fish are fixed at least 24 hours in E_1 (see under Chapter 11.8), though they can be kept in it for months. If the specimens are going to be stained, you also need alcohol + HCl, produced simply as follows: to 100 ml 70% alcohol (pure ethanol or isopropanol, not methanol), add 2 ml hydrochloric acid (HCl).

The procedure is as follows:
1. Fix in E_1 at least 24 hours
2. Transfer to 40% alcohol for two hours
3. Transfer to 50% alcohol for ten minutes
4. Transfer to borax carmine for two to five days according to thickness
5. Transfer to 50% alcohol for 30 minutes.
6. Transfer to 60% alcohol for ten minutes
7. Decolorize in alcohol + HCl for one to ten hours, according to thickness.
8. Transfer to 70% alcohol for 20 minutes.
9. Transfer to 80% alcohol for ten minutes
10. Transfer to 90% alcohol for ten minutes
11. Transfer to 95% alcohol for 15 minutes.
12. Transfer to 100% alcohol for 15 minutes, and chance once.

If shrinkage occurs when the specimen is transferred from 100% alcohol into xylol, proceed as follows:
13. Transfer to a mixture of 75% alcohol + 25% xylol for 15 minutes.
14. Transfer to a mixture of 50% alcohol + 50% xylol for 15 minutes.
15. Transfer to a mixture of 25% alcohol + 75% xylol for 15 minutes.
16. Transfer to 100% xylol for 25 minutes.
17. Imbed in balsam.

Thick worms and large arthropods stay longer in the xylol stages (up to two hours). If the inside of the specimen suddenly goes black in transmitted light or white in incident (reflected) light while being imbedded in balsam (e.g., Entellan), then more care must be taken when imbedding. Prepare a mixture of 10% balsam + 90% xylol in a small dish. Leave the specimen in that until the xylol evaporates, leaving behind a syrupy medium. Now it can be imbedded. Another way is to stab the specimen, while it soaks in the xylol, three or four times with a very fine needle. Now the balsam can penetrate and the specimen remains clear. If these suggestions do not produce translucent or transparent specimens, then proceed with methods E_3 or E_5. Practice with small worms, water fleas, and other easily obtainable microorganisms. Tapeworm segments (Photograph No. 96) are prepared by this method.

11.8.3. Permanent Mounts in Glycerin Gelatin (E₅)

This is a very gentle method of preparing specimens. It is suitable for all specimens that shrink with methods E_3 and E_4 or decolorize too much. Fix just for 24 hours in E_1 and then wash it out for two hours in 50% alcohol. Now transfer the specimen to 60% alcohol for 15 minutes, and then it can be stained for one to three days in alcohol borax carmine (Grenacher). Afterward, return it to 60% alcohol. If the stain is intensive or too deep, then it can be differentiated or cleared out by alcohol + HCl, then washed for an hour in 70% isopropyl alcohol. It remains at each of the four stages for 15 minutes (80%, 90%, 95%, and 100% isopropyl alcohol). To go further with the preparation, you need a mixture of 95 ml isopropyl alcohol (100%) plus 5 mg of glycerin, which you store in a tightly closed bottle. Pour about 5 ml of the mixture into a shallow vessel, put the specimen in it, and place it in a warm, dust-free spot. The isopropyl alcohol will evaporate and, in several hours to several days, the specimen will be in pure glycerin. The time can be regulated by the area of the surface that is evaporating or by a partial cover. Vessels with concave bottoms are very suitable, because the specimens collect at the deepest point.

The specimens can now be transferred directly from the alcohol-free glycerin right into the glycerin gelatin on a glass slide for imbedding. With a small knife or spatula, take a drop-sized piece of glycerin gelatin and center it on the slide. Heat the slide briefly in a flame. When the glycerin gelatin has melted, do not imbed the worms at once, but wait until the gelatin has cooled down somewhat. Then transfer the worms with a dissecting needle from the glycerin to the slide and place them in the glycerin gelatin. If the gelatin is already too viscous when you drop the cover slip on, you can warm the slide briefly again. Let the mount remain horizontal until the glycerin gelatin solidifies. Scrape away any excess material and seal the edges of the cover slip. The sealing operation has to be repeated during the next few days. For practice, try preparing small nematodes from the soil, vinegar worms, or microworms from food animal breeding tanks.

11.8.4. Stain Fixation of Flagellates and Ciliates (E₆)

Before flagellates and ciliates can even be tentatively identified, they must be fixed so that the cell shape, nucleus, and flagella can be recognized. A methyl green formalin solution is a suitable stain. To make a working solution, add 0.1 g methyl green and 80 ml distilled water to a brown or amber bottle that can be closed tightly. Agitate gently to dissolve the dye, then add 20 ml formalin (30 to 40%). When all the ingredients are mixed, the solution is ready for use.

For a nuclear stain, carmine-acetic acid is better suited for many flagellates, although it destroys the flagella.

We usually start with fresh preparations that contain intestinal contents, bile, or skin smears. First lift the cover slip and remove all solid, thick tissue residue. Then add some physiological saline and replace the cover slip. If the preparation is too thick, it can remain a while until the evaporation of the water in it reduces the internal space or gap. Then add a few drops of methyl green formalin along the edge of the cover slip and observe at 200 to 300X how the flagellates die. After the fluid stops swirling in the slide (caused by adding the fluid above), search out isolated specimens and observe them under maximum power.

For a uniformly distributed staining solution, place a small drop of liquid containing flagellates, or else a skin smear with very little water, on a slide. Next to that drop place a drop of methyl green formalin solution or carmine-acetic acid about a half to a quarter the size of the flagellate drop. Mix the two drops together quickly with a dissecting needle and lay a cover slip over it. Seek out, under medium power, a well-preserved flagellate, then study it under maximum power. Since protozoa fixed by this method will not keep, it is advisable to make a drawing or at least a sketch of the specimen.

Methyl green formalin stains the cell nuclei of blood and skin cells greenish blue, while the protoplasm appears pale green (Photograph No. 85). If the cells stain deep green, too much staining solution was used.

Carmine-acetic acid stains the cell nucleus red and the protoplasm pink.

11.8.5. Staining of Bacteria

Bacterial staining requires an alcohol burner, a Bunsen burner, or a propane torch, as well as a staining stand or rack that can be built of wire. The stand has to be high enough for the flame to be held briefly under it and wide enough to hold three or four slides placed side by side on it. The legs should spread to make the base broader than the platform on which the slides rest; that gives it stability. It stands in a photographic or similar tray to catch the staining solution that runs off of the slides (Photograph No. 117).

Stains are difficult to remove from household items and should not be poured down the drain or the toilet. Put used stains in tightly closed bottles and give them to the special garbage collectors who come regularly for non-standard garbage.

A layman cannot do a complete identification of bacteria, which requires growth on special culture media. The colony size, color, and other characteristics must be evaluated by experts. An alert microscopist, however, can identify the pathogens enough to determine which antibiotic can be used to fight them. For that, you have to note the appropriate size and motibility of the bacteria (Chapters 1 and 4, Chart 21). The exact size can be determined later from the fixed and stained mount.

Now make smears from the liquid that contains the bacteria. To prepare organs, squash small bits of the tissue between two clean slides. Then take a clean slide and squash it against one of the first squashed slides; take a second clean slide and do the same with it on the other of the first squashed slides. You now have four very thin squash mounts. (Tubercular cysts are also worked up in this way.) The four slides are dried in the air for about two hours. Then they have to be fixed by heat.

To fix the slides by heat, hold the slide, specimen side up, between thumb and forefinger and pass it through the flame three times. The underside of the slide must become hot enough to feel it, but not hot enough to burn you if you put it briefly on the back of your hand. (If the specimen side burns, smokes, or smells strongly the heat-fixation was too hot.) The slides are now ready.

11.8.6. Gram Stain (E₇)

Take one or more of the fixed smear slides and lay them on the staining stand to carry out the Gram staining procedure. The slides must be horizontal so that the stain does not run off. The times given in the schematic instructions may vary according to your own experience. As you pour on the stain, use the forceps, not your fingers (because the dye stains the skin deeply), to hold the slide until the carbol gentian violet solution completely covers the smear. After three minutes tilt the slide to let the staining solution run off.

As rapidly as possible, drop on potassium iodide-iodine solution, let it run off, and drop on some more. Let it act a total of 80 seconds. Let it run off and wash the slide for 60 seconds in a vessel containing spirits (94% alcohol). Let the slide drip by holding it vertically on absorbent blotting or filter paper. Then let it dry horizontally for a few minutes.

Now counterstain for 80 seconds with fuchsin solution (Gram). After thoroughly rinsing under running water, air-dry the smear, add a small drop of balsam, and lay on a cover slip. The space between the smear and the cover glass must be minimal so that you can use the oil immersion lens. If you liquify the balsam with a third of xylol, the space between cover slip and slide becomes even less.

Gram-positive bacteria appear blue violet and the Gram-negative ones red. This stain works because of the ability of the Gram-positive bacteria to keep the violet color in an alcohol bath (differentiation), while Gram-negative bacteria lose that color (Photograph No. 118), but stain red with fuchsin. If the differentiation is carried out too long, however, even the Gram-positive bacteria will lose their color, too.

11.8.7. Ziehl-Neelsen Stain (E₈)

This stain is used to identify tuberculosis bacilli. If you are uncertain whether cysts in tissues and organs are due to tuberculosis or to *Ichthyophonus,* use this stain to render the tuberculosis bacilli visible.

Old cysts often do not contain any bacteria, so several cysts must always be prepared as squash mounts.

Place the air-dried and heat-fixed specimens on the staining rack and flood the slide completely with carbol fuchsin (Ziehl-Neelsen) stain. Now heat the slide (by placing the burner flame under the slide) until fumes arise from the staining solution. Under no circumstances must the solution boil. The phenolic fumes are harmful, so work in the open or at an opened window. Keep the stain solution fuming for three minutes by warming it as needed. Replenish any evaporated staining solution to keep the smear from drying out. Then let the slide cool off for one minute and dump off the staining solution. Rinse thoroughly under running water and swish the slide around for 60 to 90 seconds in alcohol + HCl (see Chapter 11.8.2). Then rinse off again thoroughly under running water. Stain for three minutes with methylene blue solution (Loeffler) that is diluted 1:5 with distilled water. Rinse off the staining solution with distilled water and dry the slide in the air. Add a small drop of diluted balsam and cover with a cover slip.

Tuberculosis bacilli appear red, while other bacteria and tissue fragments show up blue (Photograph No. 119). To make the mount permanent, clean off the slide after it dries and seal around the cover slip.

11.8.8. Simple Bacterial Staining (E_9)

Bacteria can be stained quickly and deeply with carbol fuchsin (Ziehl-Neelsen) and with methylene blue (Loeffler). The procedure is the same for both. Unfortunately, the tissue fragments in the smear also take up the stain, thus obscuring any bacteria in them. The procedure is as follows:

1. Air-dry the smear on the slide for one to two hours;
2. Heat fix;
3. Drop on carbol fuchsin or methylene blue and let it act for five minutes;
4. Rinse under running water;
5. Air dry;
6. Imbed in diluted balsam.

Examine the mounts under 300 to 600X power.

11.8.9 Staining of Mucosa and Skin (E_{10})

Skin, blood, and many squash preparations are not very contrasty specimens. Any parasites in them are indeed easily recognizable, although the tissue structure, cellular walls, and nuclei do not stand out very much. If you want to see more details, you must stain the specimen. Methylene blue (Loeffler) is suitable, diluted 1:5 and kept in a tightly closing bottle.

Add a like quantity of the staining solution to the water on the smear on the slide or to the blood (which is diluted with physiological saline) on the slide, then wait a minute before covering with a cover slip. Blot up any excess fluid exuding from the edges of the cover slip. The cell nucleus stains deeper than the protoplasm. Less staining solution produces weaker coloration. To make the stain deeper, add the staining solution to the specimen on the slide without adding any water first. The blood smear shown in Photograph No. 40 was stained in this way. Ciliates, too, stain well with this method.

11.9. Photography as a Means of Documentation

Any microscopist occasionally comes across objects under his microscope that so please him that he wants to preserve them forever. Thus is born the wish to capture the image photographically. Another reason is that you may not be certain that the good specimen you are observing will make it undamaged out of the fresh mount once you start isolating and working with it. It is just those rare specimens that get lost easily. Well-made photographs, on the other hand, can even be helpful in identification. Many specimens are so difficult to prepare and mount that photography is the only way to document them.

No special camera is needed to produce good photomicrographs. Any single-lens reflex camera with changeble lenses is suitable. The lighting is much more important. A lot of light is necessary, and the Koehler system of illumination is absolutely necessary for first-class pictures. You can read in the instructions that come with your microscope just how to set up Koehler lighting.

Good photographs cannot be taken of a poorly prepared mount. The higher the power, the thinner must be the specimen because the depth of field or of sharp focus becomes shallower as the magnification increases.

The camera body or housing is connected to the ocular tube via a microscope adaptor, various kinds of which are on the market (Photo-

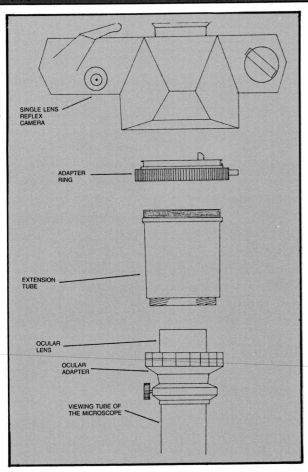

SINGLE LENS
REFLEX
CAMERA

ADAPTER
RING

EXTENSION
TUBE

OCULAR
LENS

OCULAR
ADAPTER

VIEWING TUBE OF
THE MICROSCOPE

120. Microscope adapter for 35mm camera. Universal adapter with adjustable connector.

graph No. 120). One kind, for example, slips over the upper part of the microscope tube and thus replaces the eye with a camera through the finder of which you can see the specimen and focus it by using the microscope's normal coarse and fine adjustment focusing knobs.

There are several considerations in working with a camera. Basically, any single-lens reflex is suitable for photomicrography. In practice, however, usually only models with a built-in exposure meter are used today. These "internal metering" models automatically determine the shutter speed and, in some cameras, even set it for you; in other cameras you read it from a scale in the finder and manually set the exposure with that value. With both systems, it is sometimes necessary to correct the automatically derived exposure because it represents

an average value based upon the light and the dark portions of the subject about to be photographed. This internal measuring system is built into many modern cameras. A few very new models provide spot measurement, which bases the exposure only on a small spot in the middle of the scene.

With every shot, check on the size of the specimen in comparison with the size of the photographs and whether any heavy contrast predominates. If, in brightfield shots, the specimen is darker than the background, then corrections must be made in the positive direction. In darkfield shots, on the other hand, the specimen is much lighter than the background, so correction must be in the negative direction. Since the measuring system is an average value based upon light and dark portions of the scene (or microscopic field), the exposure time must be lengthened or shortened in order to properly light the subject. The amount of correction depends upon two factors: the size of the specimen, and the difference in brightness between specimen and background. On brightfield shots the exposure time is lengthened, and in darkfield shots it is shortened.

There are only minimal differences in film quality. Many photographs today are made with films that produce color slides. The higher the ASA number or rating the grainier (or more sandy looking) the enlargements. Films between 50 and 200 ASA (or 18 to 24 DIN) are the most common. Very fine-grained films (ASA 25 or DIN 15) have longer exposure times. Many professionals work with black-and-white films because these have less grain at higher ASA ratings compared to color films.

A green filter can be used to increase the contrast in black-and-white photographs.

The color in a color photograph depends less upon the film than upon the color filter used in the microscope. This in turn depends upon the color temperature of the lighting. With non-adjustable microscope lamps, use a blue filter (B12. With adjustable lamps, use filter B9 at the brightest setting, B12 at a middle setting, and B15 with the weakest illumination.

A powerful source of light is needed for making photomicrographs with short exposure times (for motile specimens) or at high magnifications. The built-in low-voltage lamp in the larger microscopes is adequate enough for low-power viewing.

At higher magnifications the specimen should not move, so a drop of formalin or fixative stain (E_6) can be touched to the edge of one side of the cover slip and made to flow through the mount by holding a piece of blotting or filter paper on the opposite side of the cover slip, where it draws the stain across by capillary action.

At very high power, the exposure time is longer than the automatic mechanism of the camera can provide, so you have to take test shots, doubling the exposure time of each until you find an approrpriate exposure. Good photographs depends upon degree of magnification, the light intensity, and the filter, among other factors.

Microscopes provided with a mirror for illumination can be lighted with a slide projector. If the field of vision is not uniformly lighted, then place a piece of ground glass between the projector and the microscope mirror. Tracing paper also is well suited to diffuse the light.

Hardly anyone can remember the exact details of exposure once the film is processed and the pictures are ready, so it is essential to note the important facts of every exposure when it is made. This data later can be transferred to the frame of the color slide. Better yet, note this information immediately on filing cards to match each successful color slide and give both this filing card and the color slide the same number you give the protocol/autopsy card and any permanent mounts of the same specimen. Cards in the photo filing system should have the following information:

1. File number
2. Specimen name
3. Date photographed
4. Film number (if more than one)
5. Photograph number
6. Film brand
7. Film speed (ASA or DIN)
8. Correction factor
9. Microscopic magnification
10. Lamp setting
11. Filter
12. Condenser aperture setting
13. Illumination (brightfield, darkfield, phase-contrast)
14. Objective lens power
15. Ocular lens power
16. Color slide magnification
17. Size of specimen in millimeters
18. Drawing or notes on the other side

The same file number thus refers to all information on a specific specimen and makes retrieval easy.

When sending anyone color slides or prints of color or black-and-white photographs, give the actual size (in micrometers) of the specimen and not the microscopic magnification.

ACETONE: (CH₃COCH₃) is available in drug-stores and pharmacies, and from various chemical firms. The use of acetone in the tank can often lead to extensive bacterial proliferation, coating the filter with white slime and making the water turbid, leading to serious oxygen depletion and the risk of the fish suffocating if nothing is done to remedy the situation. An extensive change of water—either by adding it or by transferring the fish to it—must be done immediately.

ACRIFLAVINE: also known as 3,6-Diamino-10-methylacridinium chloride mixed with 3-6 acridinediamine, neutral acriflavine, euflavine, neutroflavine and gonacrine
An antiseptic, protozoacide and dye. Reportedly effective against *Babesia bigemina* and *B. bovis.*

ALUM: see Aluminum Potassium Sulfate

ALUMINUM POTASSIUM SULFATE: also known as alum, potassium alum and kalinite
An astringent, antiseptic and antimycotic.

AUREOMYCIN: see Chlortetracycline

BORGAL: a solution for injection, a mixture of trimethoprim and sulfadoxine. Dosage is 15 ml to 100 liters water.
> *Available*
> Hoechst Canada, Inc.
> Animal Health Dept.
> 295 Henderson Drive
> Regina, Saskatchewan
> S4N 6C2, Canada
> as Borgal

CALCIPOT: Calcium plus phosphorus and at least vitamins D and E. Works nicely bound to water-insoluble powder when vitamizing feed.
> *Available*
> Hoechst AG
> 6230 Frankfurt (Main) 80
> West Germany
> as Calcipot

CHLORAMPHENICOL: also known as chloromycetin, enicol, levomycetin, sintomycin, chlorocid, detreomycin, paraxin, chloronitrin, kemicetine, mychel, amphicol, farmecitina, tevocin, intramycetin, animycetin, synthomycin and kamycetin

A broad-spectrum antibiotic. It is active against a wide spectrum of gram-negative and gram-positive organisms, such as *Escherichia coli, Moraxella lacunata,* staphylococci including *S. aureus,* streptococci including *S. pneumoniae* and *S. hemolyticus, Proteus, Neisseria* and *Klebsiella/Enterobacter* spp. In vitro, chloramphenicol is active against the lymphogranuloma psittacosis group and *Vibrio cholerae.* Susceptible are several anaerobes, such as *Bacteroides fragilis,* as well as *Rickettsia* and *Chlamydia* spp. Of special note is the efficacy against many *Salmonella* including *S. typhi, Hemophilus influenzae* and the resistance of most strains of *Pseudomonas aeruginosa.*
> *Available:*
> Zenith Laboratories, Inc.
> 140 Legrand Avenue
> Northvale, NJ 07647 USA
> as chloramphenicol
> Parke-Davis
> Division of Warner-Lambert
> Company
> 201 Tabor Road
> Morris Plains, NJ 07950 USA
> as Chloromycetin

CHLOROMYCETIN: see Chloramphenicol

CHLORTETRACYCLINE: also known as aureomycin, biomycin and vimycin; see also Tetracyclines
A broad-spectrum antibiotic and growth stimulant. Effective against gram-positive and gram-negative bacteria, some large viruses and Rickettsiae.

COMBISONUM: an opthalmic ointment containing neomycin. If not available, neomycinsulfate can be used as bath (A₃).
> *Available*
> Hoechst AG
> 6230 Frankfurt (Main) 80
> West Germany
> as Combisonum

CONCURAT: see Tetramisole

COTRIMSTADA-FORTE: contains sulfamethoxazol and trimethoprim.
> *Available*
> Hoechst AG

6230 Frankfurt (Main) 80
West Germany
as Cotrimstada-forte

DIMETHYL SULFOXIDE: also known as DMSO, dolicur, dromisol, SQ 9453, infiltrine and domoso. Very toxic; to be avoided. A solvent, analgesic and anti-inflammatory.

DOXYCYCLINE: also known as 6-Deoxyoxytetracycline and vibramycin; see also Tetracyclines
A tetracycline antibiotic active against Rickettsiae, *Mycoplasma pneumoniae,* agents of psittacosis, ornithosis, agents of *Lymphogranuloma venereum, Granuloma inguinale,* and *Borrelia recurrentis.* The following gram-negative microorganisms are susceptible: *Haemophilus ducreyi, Pasturella pestis, P. tularensis, Bartonella bacilliformis, Bacteroides spp, Vibrio comma, V. fetus* and *Brucella* spp.

DRYLIN: see Sulfamethoxazole

DYLOX
An agricultural chemical.
Available
Mobay
8400 Hawthrone
Kansas City, MO 64130 USA

EUSAPRIM: see Sulfamethoxazole

FLAGYL: see Metronidazole

FLUBENDAZOL: also known as flumoxal and flumoxane
An anthelmintic compound (a benzimidazole) for antiparasitic use based on the prototype parent compound thiabendazole.

FLUBENOL: contains flubendazol, for which dosage is 10 mg to 5 ml acetone or DMSO per 100 liters

FORMALDEHYDE SOLUTION: formalin, formol
A disinfectant, antiseptic, astringent and embalming fluid. Used for skin infections of fish.

FORMALIN: see Formaldehyde Solution

FULVICIN: see Griseofulvin

FURAZOLIDONE: also known as furoxone, furoxane, furovag, giarlam, giardil, medaron, neftin, nicolen, nifulidone, ortazol, roptazol, tikofuran and topazone
A nitrofuran with a broad antimicrobial spectrum, including *Escherichia coli, Staphylococcus, Proteus, Salmonella, Shigella, Clostridium, Streptococcus, Eimeria, Histomonas* spp., *Aerobacter aerogenes, Vibrio cholerae* and *Giardia lamblia.*
Available:
Norwich Eaton Pharmaceuticals, Inc.
A Proctor & Gamble Company
Norwich, NY 13815-0231 USA
as Furoxone

GABBROCOL: not available in any English-speaking country

GELATIN: also known as gelfoam and puragel
For inhibiting crystals in bacteriology, for preparing cultures.
Available:
The Upjohn Company
Kalamazoo, MI 49001 USA
as Gelfoam

GRISEOFULVIN: also known as gris-PEG, grisactin, grifulvin V and fulvicin
An antifungal agent effective against common dermatophytes: *Microsporum, Epidermophyton* and *Trichophyton* spp. It has no effect on bacteria, yeasts, *Actinomyces* and *Nocardia* spp., or on other genera of fungi.
Available:
Schering Corporation
Galloping Hill Road
Kenilworth, NJ 07033 USA
as Fulvicin
Ortho Pharmaceutical Corporation
Dermatological Division
P.O. Box 300
Route 202
Raritan, NJ 08869-0602 USA
as Grifulvin V

Ayerst Laboratories
Division of American Home Products Corporation
685 Third Ave.

New York, NY 10017-4071 USA
as Grisactin

Herbert Laboratories
Dermatology Division of Allergan
Pharmaceuticals, Inc.
2525 Dupont Drive
Irvine, CA 92715 USA
as Gris-PEG

INFILTRINE: see Dimethyl Sulfoxide

MASOTEN: discontinued; see Dylox,
Trichlorfon

METRIFONATE: see Trichlorfon

METRIFORATE: see Trichlorfon

METRONIDAZOLE: also known as satric,
protostat, metryl, metric and flagyl
An antibacterial and antiprotozoal agent. It
is active against obligate anaerobes, but
apparantly does not possess clinically
relevant activity against facultative
anaerobes, obligate aerobes or
microaerophilic bacteria other than
Campylobacter fetus and *Corynebacterium
vaginalis*. At some concentrations, it is
active against *Bacteroides fragilis*, *B.
melaninogenicus*, *Fusobacterium* and
Clostridium spp. Generally less active
against non-sporeforming, gram-positive
bacilli, such as *Actinomyces*,
Propionobacterium, *Bifidobacterium* and
Eubacterium spp. It is somewhat less active
against gram-positive cocci, such as
Peptostreptococcus and *Peptococcus* spp.

Available
Searle Pharmaceuticals Inc.
Box 5110
Chicago, IL 60680 USA

as Flagyl
Schein Pharmaceutical Inc.
5 Harbor Drive
Port Washington, NY 11050 USA

as metronidazole
The Fielding Company
2384 Centerline Industrial Drive
St. Louis, MO 63146 USA

as Metric
Danbury Pharmacal, Inc.
131 West Street

P.O. Box 296
Danbury, CT 06810 USA
as metronidazole

Lederle Laboratories
Division of American Cyanamid Co.
One Cyanamid Plaza
Wayne, NY 07470 USA
as metronidazole

Zenith Laboratories, Inc.
140 Legrand Avenue
Northvale, NJ 07647 USA
as metronidazole

Lemmon Ethical Division
Lemmon Company
Sellersville, PA 18960 USA
as Metryl

Ortho Pharmaceutical Corporation
Raritan, NJ 08869 USA
as Protostat

Savage Laboratories
Division of Altana Inc.
60 Baylis Road
P.O. Box 2006
Melville, NY 11747 USA
as Satric

NEGUVON: see Trichlorfon

NEOCALCIT: a vitamin preparation. See
Calcipot.

Available
Hoechst AG
6230 Frankfurt (Main) 80
West Germany
as Neocalcit

NEOMYCIN SULFATE
A broad spectrum antibiotic. Bactericidal
notably to *Stapylococcus aureus* and
Proteus spp. Active mainly against gram-
negative organisms, except *Bacteroides*
spp. and *Pseudomonas aeruginosa* are
resistant.

Available:
Lederle Laboratories
Division of American Cyanamid Co.
One Cyanamid Plaza
Wayne, NJ 07470 USA
as neomycin sulfate

Biocraft Laboratories, Inc.
92 Route 46
Elmwood Park, NJ 07407 USA
as neomycin sulfate
Roxane Laboratories, Inc.
P.O. 16532
Columbus, OH 43216 USA
as neomycin sulfate

NITROFURANTOIN: also known as furadantin, dantafur, furagin, furazidin, furadoine, furachel and N-(5-Nitro-2-furfurylidene)-1-aminohydantoin
Susceptible organisms include *Escherichia coli, Staphylococcus aureus, Streptococcus pyogenes* and *Aerobacter aerogenes. Proteus spp., Pseudomonas aeruginosa* and *Streptococcus faecalis* are usually resistant.
Available:
Norwich Eaton Pharmaceuticals, Inc.
A Proctor & Gamble Company
Norwich, NY 13815-0231 USA
as Furadantin

Schein Pharmaceutical Inc.
5 Harbor Park Drive
Port Washington, NY 11050 USA
as nitrofurantoin

NYSTATIN: also known as nilstat and mycostatin
An antifungal and antibiotic. It is active against a variety of yeasts and yeast-like fungi. It has no appreciable activity against bacteria, actinomycetes, viruses or trichomonads.
Available:
E. R. Squibb & Sons, Inc.
General Offices
P.O. Box 4000
Princeton, NJ 08540 USA
as Mycostatin

Lederle Laboratories
Division of American Cyanamid Co.
One Cyanamid Plaza
Wayne, NJ 07470 USA
as Nilstat

Lemmon Ethical Division
Lemmon Company
Sellersville, PA 18960 USA
as nystatin

OSSPULVIT: multivitamin and trace element combination bound to a water-insoluble powder.
Available
Hoechst AG
6230 Frankfurt (Main) 80
West Germany
as Osspulvit

OXYTETRACYCLINE: also known as terramycin, imperacin, berkmycin, tetran, oxyterracin, tetrachel, liquamycin, biostat and oxysteclin; see also Tetracyclines
Active against infections caused by *Rickettsiae, Mycoplasma pneumoniae,* agents of psittacosis and ornithosis, agents of *Lymphogranuloma venereum* and *Granuloma inguinale,* and *Borrelia recurrentis.* Use against the gram-negative microorganisms *Haemophilus ducreyi, Pasturella pestis, P. tularensis, Bartonella bacilliformis, Bacteroides* spp., *Vibrio comma, V. fetus* and *Brucella* spp.
Available:
Pfipharmecs Division
Pfizer Inc.
235 East 42nd Street
New York, NY 10017 USA
as Terramycin

PIPERAZINE CITRATE: also known as antepar, tripiperazine dicitrate, multifuge, oxucide, pipizan citrate, pinrou, exopin, parazine, helmezine and arpezine
Piperazine, along with its derivative diethylcarbamazine, is an anthelmintic. The spectrum of activity is largely against ascarid parasites in all species and also *Oesophagostomum* spp. There is a variable activity against hookworms and strongyles, but little effect against whipworms or flatworms.
Available
Burroughs Wellcome Co.
3030 Cornwallis Road
Research Triangle Park, NC 27709 USA
as Antepar

QUININE SULFATE: also known as quinamm and quindam
A neuromuscular agent, more toxic than

quinine hydrochloride. See C$_4$.

Available:
Merrell Dow Pharmaceuticals Inc.
Subsidiary of The Dow Chenical
Company
Cincinnati, OH 45242-9553 USA
as Quinamm

Danbury Pharmacal, Inc.
131 West Stret
P.O. Box 296
Danbury, CT 06810 USA
as Quindam

Zenith Laboratories, Inc.
140 Legrand Avenue
Northvale, NJ 07647 USA
as quinine sulfate

Lederle Laboratories
Division of American Cyanamid Co.
One Cyanamid Plaza
Wayne, NJ 07470 USA
as quinine sulfate

Schein Pharmaceutical Inc.
5 Harbor Park Drive
Port Washington, NY 11050 USA
as quinine sulfate

SULFAMETHOXAZOLE: also known as gantanol, gantonol, sulfasomezole, sulfamethylisoxazole, sulfamethoxiazole and sinomin; see also Sulfonamides
A sulfonamide.

Available:
Roche Laboratories
Division of Hoffmann-La Roche Inc.
Nutley, NJ 07110 USA
as Gantanol

SULFATHIAZOLE: also known as norsulfazol, 2090 RP, M & B 760, duatok, avisol and 2-Sulfanylaminothiazole; see also Sulfonamides
An antimicrobial and sulfonamide.

SULFONAMIDES: widey used antibacterial agents in veterinary medicine. The sulfonamides include sulfamethazine, sulfabromethazine, sulfadimethoxidine, sulfathiazole, sulfamethoxazole, sulfadoxine, sulfamethazine, sulfadiazine, sulfaquinoxaline, sulfadimethoxine, sulfaethoxypyridazine, sulfapyridine and succinylsulfathiazole and others. The synergistic action of sulfonamides with trimethoprim has broadened sulfonamide therapy.

TERRAMYCIN: see Oxytetracycline

TETRACYCLINE: also known as achromycin, tetracyn, hostacycline, panmycin, bristacycline, polyotic, steclin, solvodin and criseocycline; see also Tetracylines
A broad spectrum antibiotic indicated for infections caused by the following microorganisms: *Rickettsiae, Mycoplasma pneumoniae,* agents of psittacosis and ornithosis, agents of *Lymphogranuloma venereum* and *Granuloma inguinale,* and *Borrelia recurrentis.* It is effective against the gram-negative microorganisms *Haemophilus ducreyi, Pasturella pestis, P. tularensis, Bartonella bacilliformis, Brucella* and *Bacteroides* spp., *Vibrio comma* and *V. fetus.*

Available:
Parke-Davis
Division of Warner-Lambert Co.
201 Tabor Road
Morris Plains, NJ 07950 USA
as tetracylcine HCI

TETRACYCLINES Very broad-spectrum antibiotics with similar antimicrobial features. They differ somewhat from one another in their spectra and pharmacokinetic fates. There are three naturally occurring tetracyclines (oxytetracycline, chlortetracycline and demethylchlortetracycline). Several are derived semisynthetically (tetracycline, rolitetracycline, methacycline, minocycline, doxycycline, lymecycline and others).

TETRAMISOLE: also known as tetramizole, nilverm, ripercol, citarin, concurat, galinid, anthelvet, decaris, R 8299, McN-JR 8299, Bayer 9051, ICI 50,627 and d1-2,3,5,6-Tetrahydro-6phenylimidazo [2,1-b] thiazole
An anthelmintic.

TRIAMCINOLONE ACETONIDE: also known as kenolog, vetalog and ledercort - D, orion, volon and cinonide

An adrenocorticosteroid, glucocorticoid and antiinflammatory.
Available:
Legere Pharmaceuticals, Inc.
7326 E. Evans Road
Scottsdale, AZ 85260 USA
as cinonide

TRICAINE: also known as MS-222, ethyl-m-aminobenzoate methanesulfonate and metacaine
An anesthetic and narcotic. It is one of the safest anesthetics for fish. Lower dosages tranquilize. Following its use, large numbers of fish can be transported in a limited amount of water with supplemental oxygen. Solutions are toxic to fish if used in direct sunlight or salt water. Do not use within three weeks of harvesting fish for human consumption.

TRICHLORFON: also known as neguvon, dipterex, ditrifon, dylox, dyrex, dyvon, chlorphos, chlorofos, metrifonate, trichlorophon(e), Bot-X, hypodix, wotexit, delicia, Bayer L 13/59, anthon and 0-0-Dimethyl 2,2,2-trichloro-1-hydroxyethyl phosphonate
An insecticide.

TRICHLORPHON: see Trichlorfon

TRIMETHOPRIM: also known as monotrim, proloprim, syraprim, tiempe, trimanyl, trimopan, trimpex and wellcoprim
Used alone, this diaminopyrimidine is not particularly effective against bacteria. The combination of trimethoprim and sulfonamides has expanded sulfonamide therapy. The synergistic action is effective against gram-negative and gram-positive organisms, including *Actinomyces, Bordetalla, Clostridium, Corynebacterium, Fusobacterium, Haemophilus, Klebsiella, Pasteurella, Proteus, Salmonella, Shigella* and *Campylobacter* spp, as well as *Escherichia coli, Streptococci* and *Staphylococci. Pseudomonas* and *Mycobacterium* spp. are not susceptible.
Available:
Biocraft Laboratories, Inc.
92 Route 46
Elmwood Park, NJ 07407 USA
as trimethoprim

Danbury Pharmacal, Inc.
131 West Street
P.O. Box 296
Danbury, CT 06810 USA
as trimethoprim

TRYPAFLAVINE: see Acriflavine

VIBRAMYCIN: see Doxycycline

VOLON: see Triamcinolone Acetonide

VMP: not available in any English-speaking country

GENERAL INDEX

Index to Photos